Thyroid and Parathyroid Disorders in Children

Thyroid and Parathyroid
Disorders in Children

Thyroid and Parathyroid Disorders in Children

A Practical Handbook

Edited by

Pallavi Iyer and Herbert Chen

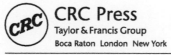

CRC Press
Taylor & Francis Group
Boca Raton London New York

CRC Press is an imprint of the
Taylor & Francis Group, an **informa** business

First edition published 2021
by CRC Press
6000 Broken Sound Parkway NW, Suite 300, Boca Raton, FL 33487-2742

and by CRC Press
2 Park Square, Milton Park, Abingdon, Oxon, OX14 4RN

ISBN: 9780367555436 (hbk)
ISBN: 9780367419868 (pbk)
ISBN: 9780367419875 (ebk)

Typeset in Minion
by Deanta Global Publishing Services, Chennai, India

Dedication

We would like to dedicate this book to the wonderful patients and their families who inspire us.

Contents

Preface

The care of a pediatric patient with a rare condition depends on thoughtful and specialized attention. The medical team often relies on clinical and educational multidisciplinary conferences or tumor boards to gather differing perspectives for the care of patients with complex endocrine conditions to offer family-centered recommendations. It is in this spirit that the idea for this book originated between a surgeon and an endocrinologist. The best care is delivered through a collaborative effort between patient, family members, pediatric endocrinologists, and endocrine/general/pediatric/otolaryngology surgeons along with expertise from radiologists and pathologists. *Thyroid and Parathyroid Disorders in Children: A Practical Handbook* is designed to offer an approach to diagnosing and treating children with thyroid and parathyroid diseases from international experts in the medical and surgical fields. This handbook is intended for in-training and practicing physicians, physician extenders, and other professional health care workers who care for these children and their families. It provides necessary information for a practical approach to diagnostic and therapeutic interventions in the management of thyroid and parathyroid diseases. Special attention is given to discussing differences in the recognition and management of children compared with adults.

The book is divided into two sections: thyroid and parathyroid. Before delving into specific disorders, each section discusses the use of the laboratory testing and radiographic modalities in the study of the thyroid and the parathyroid gland. This helps guide the reader in knowing the utility and limitations of each of the laboratory and radiographic findings when approaching a child with these conditions. Both common and rare disorders are described along with medical treatments and surgical techniques. We hope that the easy readability of each of these stand-alone chapters leads to this book being a reference when faced with a child with clinical symptoms concerning any of these diseases. The tables and figures in these chapters are especially helpful for quick visual review or understanding of the condition.

We are indebted to our colleagues who authored each of the chapters. We are in awe of the esteemed, world-renowned experts and upcoming future leaders for sacrificing their valuable time and sharing their expertise in creating this handbook. We also thank our students and fellows who push us to teach complex concepts in understandable and practical ways. It is our sincere hope that our readers will find these chapters clear and use this book in guiding best care of children with endocrine disorders.

Herb Chen, MD
Pallavi Iyer, MD

Acknowledgments

We are grateful to Elizabeth Chen for the design of the cover.

Editors

Pallavi Iyer

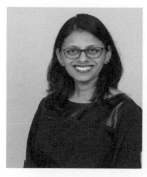

Dr. Pallavi Iyer earned her BS from The Ohio State University with a Distinction in Molecular Genetics and Honors in Liberal Arts. She graduated from medical school from The Ohio State University College of Medicine and Public Health in 2001 and finished her pediatric residency, chief residency, and pediatric endocrine fellowship at the University of South Florida. She went on to become the first medical director of a new pediatric endocrine division at Johns Hopkins All Children's Hospital in Saint Petersburg, Florida. Her interest in care for children with pediatric endocrine tumors and long-term endocrine follow-up of pediatric cancer survivors stems from taking care of patients with these unique needs. She is currently an Associate Professor of Pediatrics at the University of Alabama at Birmingham and Director of the Pediatric Thyroid Nodule Clinic. In this role, Dr. Iyer established the only interdisciplinary program dedicated to caring for children with thyroid nodule/thyroid cancer in the state of Alabama. She lives with her husband, a software developer, and her twin teenage boys in Homewood, Alabama.

Herbert Chen

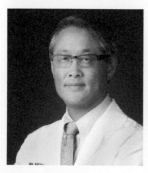

Dr. Herbert Chen earned his BS from Stanford University with Honors and with Distinction in 1988 and graduated from Duke University School of Medicine Alpha Omega Alpha in 1992. Dr. Chen then completed a general surgery residency followed by a surgical oncology and endocrinology fellowship at the Johns Hopkins Hospital. Dr. Chen is Chair of the Department of Surgery at University of Alabama at Birmingham (UAB), and the Surgeon-in-Chief of UAB Hospital and Health System. He is a Professor of Surgery and Biomedical Engineering and holds the Fay Fletcher Kerner Endowed Chair. His clinical interests include endocrine surgery, and he is a pioneer in radio-guided parathyroid surgery. Dr. Chen is the Editor-in-Chief of the *American Journal of Surgery* and serves on many other editorial boards. He is also the President of the Society of Asian Academic Surgeons Foundation, President of Surgical Biology Club II, Past-President of the Association for Academic Surgery, Past-President of the Society of Clinical Surgery, and Past-President of the American Association of Endocrine Surgeons. Dr. Chen has been recognized for his passion for teaching and mentoring the next generation of surgical leaders. Dr. Chen and his wife Harriet, a freelance photographer, reside in Mountain Brook, Alabama. His son Alex is a medical student at Yale University while his daughter Liz is a graduate student at North Carolina State University.

List of Contributors

Ambika P. Ashraf, MD, FAAP
Division of Pediatric Endocrinology
and Diabetes
Metabolic Bone Clinic
University of Alabama at Birmingham
Birmingham, Alabama

Erin Partington Buczek, MD
Department of Otolaryngology
University of Alabama at Birmingham
Birmingham, Alabama

Andrew C. Calabria, MD
Division of Endocrinology and
Diabetes
Center for Bone Health
The Children's Hospital of
Philadelphia
Perelman School of Medicine
University of Pennsylvania
Philadelphia, Pennsylvania

Herbert Chen, MD
University of Alabama at
Birmingham (UAB)
UAB Hospital and Health System
O'Neal Comprehensive Cancer
Center at UAB
Birmingham, Alabama

Jesse T. Davidson IV, MD
Washington University School of
Medicine
Department of Surgery
St. Louis, Missouri

Alicia Diaz-Thomas, MD, MPH
LeBonheur Children's Hospital
University of Tennessee Health
Science Center
Division of Pediatric Endocrinology
Memphis, Tennessee

Grace C. Dougan, MD
Pediatric Endocrine Associates of
Tampa, Florida
Tampa, Florida

Sophie Dream, MD
Department of Surgery
Medical College of Wisconsin
Milwaukee, Wisconsin

Jessica Fazendin, MD
Department of Surgery
University of Alabama at Birmingham
Birmingham, Alabama

Rajshri M. Gartland, MD MPH
Department of Surgery
Massachusetts General Hospital
Boston, Massachusetts

Pallavi Iyer, MD, FAAP
University of Alabama at
Birmingham (UAB)
Division of Pediatric Endocrinology
and Diabetes
Director, Thyroid Nodule Clinic
Birmingham, Alabama

Jennifer H. Kuo, MD, FACS
Thyroid Biopsy Program
Endocrine Surgery Research Program
Columbia University Medical Center
New York, New York

James A. Lee, MD
New York Thyroid-Parathyroid Center
Adrenal center
CollectedMedEducation Project
Columbia University Medical Center
New York, New York

Anne M. Lenz, MD
Pediatric Endocrine Associates of
    Tampa Florida
Tampa, Florida

Michael A. Levine, MD
Division of Endocrinology and
    Diabetes
The Children's Hospital of Philadelphia
Director, Center for Bone Health
Professor of Pediatrics and Medicine
Perelman School of Medicine at
    University of Pennsylvania
Philadelphia, Pennsylvania

Diana Lin, MD
Anatomic Pathology
University of Alabama at Birmingham
Birmingham, Alabama

Brenessa Lindeman, MD, MEHP, FACS
University of Alabama at Birmingham
UAB General Surgery Residency
Associate Designated Institutional
    Official
UAB Graduate Medical Education
Birmingham, Alabama

Haggi Mazeh, MD, FACS, FISA
Endocrine and General Surgery
Hadassah-Hebrew University Medical
    Center, Mount Scopus
Jerusalem, Israel

Catherine McManus, MD, MS
Columbia University Medical Center
Endocrine Surgery Fellow
New York, New York

Gail Mick, MD
University of Alabama at Birmingham
Division of Pediatric Endocrinology
    and Diabetes
Director, Endocrine Newborn
    Screening Clinic
Birmingham, Alabama

Todd D. Nebesio, MD
Indiana University School of Medicine
Riley Hospital for Children
Division of Pediatric Endocrinology/
    Diabetology
Indianapolis, Indiana

Kimberly Ramonell
Emory University Department of
    Surgery
Atlanta, Georgia

Scott A. Rivkees, MD
Department of Pediatrics
University of Florida
Gainesville, Florida

Allen W. Root, MD
Department of Pediatrics
Johns Hopkins University
Johns Hopkins All Children's
    Hospital
Saint Petersburg, Florida

Jessica Schmitt, MD
University of Alabama at Birmingham
Division of Pediatric Endocrinology
    and Diabetes
Birmingham, Alabama

Tracy S. Wang, MD, MPH
Section of Endocrine Surgery
Medical College of Wisconsin
Milwaukee, Wisconsin

Tal Yalon, MD
Department of General and
    Oncological Surgery – Surgery C,
Chaim Sheba Medical Center
Tel Hashomer, Ramat Gan, Israel

1

Laboratory evaluation of thyroid function

JESSICA SCHMITT AND DIANA LIN

BACKGROUND

The hypothalamic–pituitary–thyroid (HPT) axis is responsible for the regulation and production of thyroid hormone (TH). The hypothalamus secretes thyrotropin-releasing hormone (TRH), which stimulates the pituitary gland to produce thyroid-stimulating hormone (TSH), which causes the production and release of thyroid hormones (TH). The two forms of TH are thyroxine (T4) and triiodothyronine (T3). When children present with symptoms of hypothyroidism, hyperthyroidism, goiter, or thyroid nodules, in addition to a thorough history and physical, they warrant assessment of the biochemical status of the HPT axis.

At this time, clinically available tests allow for measurement of the concentration of TSH, total T3, total T4, unbound or free T4 (FT4) and free T3 (FT3), and reverse T3. In addition, antibodies associated with thyroid pathology can be detected.

AVAILABLE LABORATORY TESTS OF THYROID FUNCTION

In the majority of clinical situations, TSH and FT4 or total T4 will be sufficient to screen for common thyroid disorders such as hypothyroidism and hyperthyroidism (1). As with all tests, there can be false-negative and false-positive results. There are numerous reports in the literature describing cases in which patients were adversely affected by acting on inaccurate lab results. Before ordering or interpreting tests of thyroid function, clinicians should have an understanding of the limitations of these assays. Accurate measurement and interpretation are paramount to clinical care, and interest in this area is large. Between 1981 and 2017, over 100 articles were published discussing laboratory evaluation of thyroid status (2)! In this section, we will summarize the assays most common in clinical practice and their limitations.

When assessing thyroid function, lab tests can be categorized into those that assess the HPT axis: TSH, FT3, FT4, total T3, total T4, and reverse T3, and those that assess for autoantibodies that can affect thyroid function: thyroid peroxidase antibody (anti-TPO), thyroglobulin antibody (TgAb), and TSH receptor antibodies. TSH receptor antibodies can be inhibitory, stimulatory, or neutral. In the past, estimation of free TH concentrations relied upon resin uptake, FT4 index, and T4/thyroid binding globulin ratio (3). With increased availability and specificity of FT3 and FT4 testing, these prior tests are no longer recommended for first-line testing and they will not be discussed in this review.

TYPES OF ASSAYS USED

Immunoassays are the mainstay for measuring TSH and TH. Immunoassays rely upon a labeled antibody reacting with an analyte (such as TSH) of interest. Advantages of immunoassays include their ability to detect small amounts of analyte, lack of significant personnel oversight/participation, and quick time to result (2). As specificity of the labeled antibodies improved, so did the sensitivity of the assays. For example, the first generation TSH assays had a lower limit of detection of 1.0 mIU/L. The third generation TSH assays now have a detection of 0.01 mIU/L (1). Both biotin and streptavidin are commonly used in these immunoassays (2, 4), and this will become important when considering assay interference.

There are several forms of immunoassays relevant to thyroid evaluation:

1. Sandwich immunoassay (also known as a two-site, non-competitive immunoassay): The patient's serum is mixed with two antibodies. The "capture" antibody binds to one part of the analyte. The "labeled detector" antibody binds to another part of the analyte (1). The detector antibody measured is directly proportional to the amount of analyte present. See Figure 1.1.
2. One-step competitive immunoassay: The analyte and labeled analyte analog compete for binding to the capture assay. The amount of signal (label) detected is inversely proportional to the amount of analyte present (1). See Figure 1.2.

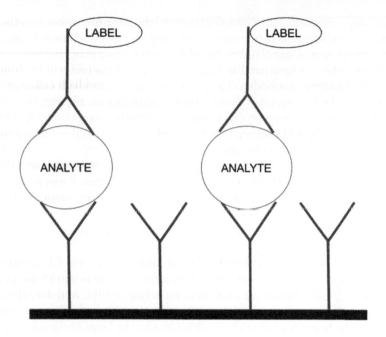

Figure 1.1 Sandwich assay.

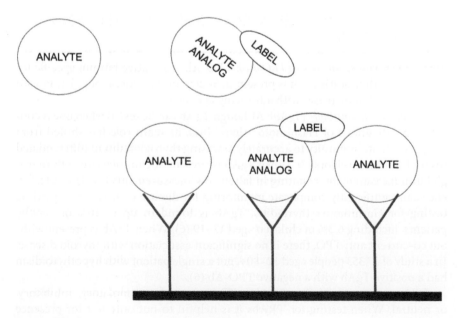

Figure 1.2 One-step competitive assay.

3. One-step non-competitive immunoassay: A labeled antibody binds to the analyte. The sample is then washed, removing the unbound labeled antibodies. The amount of signal is directly related to the amount of analyte.
4. Bioassay: This is a functional assay used to check for the presence of stimulatory TSH receptor antibodies. The patient serum is mixed with cells designed to express the TSH receptor. If stimulatory antibodies are present, they stimulate the TSH receptor, causing increased production of cyclic AMP. The amount of cyclic AMP is then measured and is proportional to the amount of stimulatory TSH receptor antibodies (1, 5).
5. Bridge-immunoassay: This two-step assay relies upon the binding of TSH receptor antibodies to both an immobilized capture receptor and a signal receptor (1, 5). The TSH receptor antibody forms a "bridge" between the capture receptor and the signal receptor. The amount of signal measured is proportional to the amount of TSH receptor antibodies present.

Measuring free hormone concentration: When measuring FT3 or FT4 concentration, one must consider the potential of measuring protein-bound T4 and T3 interacting with the capture antibody and impacting results. To reduce this, one can separate the protein-bound T3 and T4 from the FT3 and FT4 prior to measurement. The two ways to do this are ultrafiltration and equilibrium dialysis. In ultrafiltration, the sample is centrifuged and the ultrafiltrate is then measured (1). In equilibrium dialysis, there is a dialysis membrane which separates the small molecules (FT3 or FT4) from the larger molecules (proteins), allowing for direct measurement of free hormone concentrations (1).

TESTS OF ANTIBODIES ASSOCIATED WITH THYROID DYSFUNCTION

Thyroid peroxidase antibody (TPO-Ab): TPO-Ab is sensitive but not specific for Hashimoto's thyroiditis (3). It is present in 5–20% of the general population with an incidence that increases with advancing age (6).

Thyroglobulin antibody (TgAb): Although TgAb can be tested when one is considering a diagnosis of Hashimoto's thyroiditis, its main role has shifted from diagnosing autoimmunity to accurately assessing thyroglobulin in differentiated thyroid cancer survivors (3). When TgAb is present, it can interfere with thyroglobulin measurement, resulting in falsely low measurements (7). This interference can significantly complicate monitoring for disease recurrence. Regarding testing for Hashimoto's thyroiditis, TgAb is found in up to 10% of healthy patients, including 6.3% of children aged 12–19 (6). When TgAb is present without co-current anti-TPO, there is no significant association with thyroid disease. In a study of 17,353 people aged 12–80+, not a single patient with hypothyroidism had a positive TgAb with a negative TPO-Ab (6).

TSH receptor antibodies (TRAbs): TRAbs can be stimulatory, inhibitory, or neutral. When testing for TRAbs it is helpful to not only test for presence or absence, but also test for biochemical effect. All TRAbs can be detected by competitive TSH-binding assays (3), but to specifically assess for the presence of stimulatory TRAbs, the specific thyroid-stimulating-immunoglobulin (TSI) bioassay is ideal (1, 3, 5).

LIMITATIONS IN COMMON IMMUNOASSAYS

All antibody-based immunoassays are subject to potential interference. At its worst, immunoassay interference has been known to lead to unnecessary interventions, including chemotherapy and surgery (8). See Table 1.1 for common interferences in laboratory assessment of thyroid function.

Understanding laboratory interference is essential when interpreting labs assessing thyroid status. In a review of >150 case reports of interference in thyroid function tests, 50% had a documented clinical consequence (2). Consequences ranged from mild to severe, including delaying the diagnosis of thyroid storm (2).

Macro-TSH: Macro-TSH is a large biologically inactive complex of TSH and anti-TSH antibodies (2). Given its large size, it is not excreted and accumulates in the serum. Different assay platforms are more or less sensitive to macro-TSH, and values will vary based on platform used, but all available sandwich immunometric assays used to measure TSH also detect macro-TSH. This leads to falsely elevated TSH results in up to 2% of the population with these anti-TSH antibodies (2, 9). Results can range from mildly elevated to significantly elevated with concentrations >400 mIU/L (9). One should consider macro-TSH interference when the measured TSH concentration is elevated but the measured TH (FT4 or total T4) is in the upper half of the normal range (2). Of note, macro-TSH does cross the placenta, and has been shown to affect newborn screening results (10).

Biotin (vitamin B7)

The recommended daily dietary intake of biotin for children is 5 to 25 **mcg** and for adults is 30 **mcg**. Many supplements contain significantly more biotin with doses as high as 5 to 20 **mg** per dose (4). Supplementation with biotin doses as low as 1.5 mg per day have been found to affect laboratory assays (2). Biotin interferes with immunoassays by irreversibly binding to streptavidin (2, 4, 11).

Table 1.1 Interferences affecting laboratory assessment of thyroid function

Interfering element	Frequency
Macro-TSH	Common
Biotin	Common
Endogenous antibodies including:	
1. Anti-streptavidin antibodies	1.Rare
2. Anti-ruthenium (15) antibodies	2. Rare
3. Thyroid hormone autoantibodies (THAAbs)	3. Rare
4. Heterophile antibodies, human anti-mouse antibodies (16), and human anti-animal antibodies (HAAA)	4. Common

In sandwich assays using a biotin-streptavidin complex, the capture antibody is biotinylated. This biotinylated capture antibody binds to streptavidin microparticles on the assay plate (4). In samples with high plasma biotin concentrations, streptavidin microparticles on the assay plate are saturated with biotin and the capture antibody-analyte-labeled antibody sandwich gets washed away, resulting in a falsely low measurement (4).

In competitive immunoassays using a biotin-streptavidin complex, the capture antibody is biotinylated. The analyte and the labeled analyte analog compete for binding to the biotinylated capture antibody which then again binds to streptavidin microparticles on the assay plate (4). As in sandwich assays, in plasma with high biotin concentrations, the biotin will bind to the streptavidin microparticle, resulting in less capture antibody-labeled analyte binding. In this assay where the signal is inversely related to the analyte's concentration, high plasma biotin will decrease the signal detected, causing a falsely elevated result (2, 4).

As TSH is measured by a sandwich assay and FT4 by a competitive assay, biotin interference results in a falsely low TSH and falsely elevated FT4. Biotin interference should therefore be suspected in patients whose clinical history and exam are not consistent with hyperthyroidism (11).

Endogenous antibodies: Accurate antibody-based immunoassays require the interaction between the antibody and target epitope and then the binding of the analyte-antibody complex to the assay plate. Anything that interferes with these binding sites, such as biotin as explained above, can impact the test results. Endogenous antibodies affect immunoassays by interfering with the binding of the capture antibody to the analyte, the analyte to the labeled antibody, or the capture antibody to the assay plate.

Anti-streptavidin antibodies: The biotin–streptavidin interaction is essential for accurate use of many commercial labs. There are case reports of patients with anti-streptavidin antibodies leading to inaccurate tests of thyroid function but the incidence is much lower than other interferences (2, 12).

Thyroid hormone antibodies: In less than 2% of the population, adults without thyroid disease can have anti-T3 or anti-T4 antibodies (13). These anti-TH antibodies can bind to both the analyte (T3 or T4) and the capture antibody, affecting results in one-step assays. In tests that separate the analyte from the serum (two-step assays, equilibrium dialysis, and ultrafiltration), these antibodies do not affect results (2, 13, 14).

Anti-ruthenium (15) antibodies: These antibodies are present in less than 1% of the population (2) and only impact results of platforms using ruthenium.

Heterophile antibodies, human anti-mouse antibodies (16), and human anti-animal antibodies (HAAAs): These are one of the more prevalent antibodies that affect assessment of the HPT axis in clinical practice. They can impact up to 6% of the population and impact immunoassays by binding to the antibodies used in the assay (2). The more antibodies used in an assay, the more likely they are to be impacted by these antibodies. For example, most TSH immunoassays are sandwich assays, using two antibodies, and are more sensitive to antibody interference than assays for FT4 or FT3 which use only one antibody (2).

AVOIDING AND CORRECTING FOR IMMUNOASSAY INTERFERENCE

Macro-TSH: As all available TSH assays detect macro-TSH, running the sample on a different platform assay will not avoid macro-TSH interference completely. However, as different assay platforms have different sensitivity for macro-TSH, running the sample on two different platforms can suggest assay interference if the results are significantly discordant (17). If macro-TSH is suspected, the serum can be diluted or treated with polyethylene glycol (PEG) which causes large-molecular-weight proteins, including macro-TSH, to precipitate (2, 9, 17). Although these are both options, there is no clear cut-off or consensus on threshold for interpreting diluted or post-polyethylene glycol-treated serum. While dilution and treatment with PEG are reasonable screening tests, the ideal way to assess for macro-TSH interference is to measure macro-TSH directly with gel filtration chromatography (GFC) (9). As both macro-TSH and HAMA have a similar molecular weight, before doing GFC, one should treat the sample with HAMA blockers (9). Limitations to GFC testing for macro-TSH include availability and cost (17).

Biotin (vitamin B7): The simplest way to avoid biotin interference is to stop biotin supplementation for a few days before blood is drawn (2, 4). If this is not possible, one can run the sample on a non-biotin-dependent platform.

Endogenous antibodies: For anti-streptavidin and anti-Ru antibodies, running the assay on a platform that does not use streptavidin or ruthenium will eliminate the interference. For heterophile antibodies, HAMAs, and HAAAs one can repeat the assay after serial dilution, treat the sample with mouse immunoglobulin, run the assay on a different platform, or treat the sample with heterophile binders (2).

If the results of thyroid laboratory evaluation do not fit the clinical picture, one should contact one's laboratory medicine colleagues to discuss best testing options.

TESTING THYROID FINE NEEDLE ASPIRATION SPECIMENS

Although the prevalence of thyroid nodules is much lower in the pediatric population than in adults (18), these nodules are associated with a five times greater risk of malignancy (19). Fine needle aspiration (FNA) is an important tool in the management of thyroid nodules. The Bethesda System for Thyroid Cytopathology (20) defines diagnostic categories (Table 1.2). Categories III (atypia of undetermined significance) and IV (suspicious for follicular/Hürthle cell neoplasm) are considered *indeterminate* since the nodule cannot be definitively reported as benign or malignant.

Table 1.2 Bethesda System for thyroid cytopathology

Category	Diagnosis
I	Unsatisfactory/non-diagnostic
II	Benign
III	Atypia of undetermined significance/follicular lesion of undetermined significance
IV	Suspicious for follicular/Hürthle cell neoplasm
V	Suspicious for malignancy
VI	Malignant

Molecular testing

Although molecular testing is accepted for adult indeterminate nodules, these tests have not been thoroughly studied in pediatric populations. A positive mutation test is highly associated with malignancy. However, a negative test must be interpreted with caution due to the higher prevalence of malignancy for pediatric indeterminate nodules when compared to adults: Approximately 28% for Category III nodules and 35% for Category IV nodules (18). Currently the American Thyroid Association does not recommend molecular testing for routine pediatric clinical practice. Instead, the next recommended step for indeterminate nodules is surgery (18). However, molecular testing can be helpful if specific alternations identified in pediatric populations are found. Just as in adults, the BRAFV600E mutation is strongly associated with classical papillary thyroid carcinoma. *RET/PTC1* has been associated with more aggressive variants of papillary thyroid carcinoma (19).

Four molecular assays are commercially available, but, at the time of publication, none have been validated for patients under age 21 years (15, 19, 21–23).

Gene expression classifier/gene sequencing classifier (GEC/GSC): This test uses a microarray to evaluate messenger RNA (mRNA) signatures from 167 genes. One commercially available assay uses this technology, the Afirma Gene Expression Classifier. These mRNA profiles are proprietary and not reported in the test results. For a successful assay, two dedicated FNA passes should be placed in the nucleic acid preservative medium. The sample first undergoes a 25-gene assay to look for mRNA profiles associated with medullary thyroid carcinoma, parathyroid tissue, and metastatic tumors. If positive, the test is reported. If negative, the sample undergoes a 142-gene assay, and results are reported as "benign" or "suspicious." Suspicious samples undergo additional testing to identify the presence or absence of the BRAFV600E mutation. The newly developed gene sequencing classifier has improved RNA transcriptome analysis and more accurate classification of Hürthle cell lesions. Additional parameters include identifying samples with low follicular content and reporting RET/PTC fusions (21). However, a "benign" GEC result may not be truly benign in a child. Likewise, a "suspicious, BRAF negative" result does not report what gene or genes were identified in the panel, and should best be interpreted as "still indeterminate."

Targeted next-generation sequencing (NGS) tests report a risk of malignancy based on genotypes identified. Although the risk of malignancy is based on adult studies, mutations identified may be clinically useful if studied in pediatric populations. Two tests are commercially available: ThyroSeq and ThyGenX/ThyraMIR.

ThyroSeq version 3 identifies alterations in 112 genes (22). This test requires 1–2 drops from the first FNA pass or a subsequent dedicated FNA pass in nucleic acid preservative medium. If no sample was collected at the time of FNA, cell block preparations or formalin fixed paraffin embedded tissue may be used. First, the test identifies the cellular composition of the sample: Follicular cells, C-cells, parathyroid, or non-thyroid. Next, the sample undergoes sequencing analysis, and the Genomic Classifier applies a score to the sample (22). Specific genotypes are reported if identified, and the associated adult population risk of malignancy is reported. If no mutations or fusions are identified, the test is reported as "negative/low risk."

ThyGenX/ThyraMIR is a two-part test that requires one dedicated FNA pass in nucleic acid preservative medium. First, the ThyGenX test performs targeted NGS for eight genes (*BRAF V600E, RET-PTC1/3, PIC3CA, BRAF K601E, H/K/N-RAS, PAX8-PPARgamma*). The expanded panel (*ThyGeNEXT*) also includes *ALK, RET, TERT* promoter, *GNAS*, and *PTEN* (23). If positive, the genotype is reported with the associated adult risk of malignancy. If negative, the sample undergoes the second test, quantitative real-time polymerase chain reaction (ThyraMIR). ThyraMIR tests expression levels of micro RNA, small non-coding RNA that modulates mRNA to regulate gene expression. miRNA is more stable than mRNA (24). Results from this 10 miRNA classifier are reported as "high-risk" and "low-risk" by a proprietary algorithm (23).

FNA cytology smear testing is provided by the RosettaGX Reveal. One cellular direct smear is provided for nucleic acid extraction. The sample undergoes a classifier of 24 miRNA sequences, 6 of which overlap with the ThyraMIR panel (24). Results are reported as "suspicious for malignancy" or "benign" (15). Since all the diagnostic material is removed from the slide, whole-slide imaging must be performed prior to nucleic acid extraction. This is currently the only assay that tests directly visualized abnormal cells. However, microRNA signatures are an emerging area of research and have not yet been studied in pediatric thyroid carcinoma.

REFERENCES

1. Nerenz R. Thyroid Function Testing. Clinical Chemical Trainee Council, 2017.
2. Favresse J, Burlacu M-C, Maiter D, Gruson D. Interferences With Thyroid Function Immunoassays: Clinical Implications and Detection Algorithm. *Endocr Rev* 2018;39(5):830–50.

3. Soh S-B, Aw T-C. Laboratory Testing in Thyroid Conditions - Pitfalls and Clinical Utility. *Ann Lab Med* 2019;39(1):3.

4. Rosner I, Rogers E, Maddrey A, Goldberg DM. Clinically Significant Lab Errors due to Vitamin B7 (Biotin) Supplementation: A Case Report Following a Recent FDA Warning. *Cureus* 2019;11(8):e5470.

5. Allelein S, Diana T, Ehlers M, Kanitz M, Hermsen D, Schott M, Kahaly GJ. Comparison of a Bridge Immunoassay with Two Bioassays for Thyrotropin Receptor Antibody Detection and Differentiation. *Hormone Metab Res* 2019;51(06):341–6.

6. Hollowell JG, Staehling NW, Flanders WD, Hannon WH, Gunter EW, Spencer CA, Braverman LE. Serum TSH, T4, and Thyroid Antibodies in the United States Population (1988 to 1994): National Health and Nutrition Examination Survey (NHANES III). *J Clin Endocrinol Metab* 2002;87(2):489–99.

7. D'Aurizio F, Metus P, Ferrari A, Caruso B, Castello R, Villalta D, et al. Definition of the Upper Reference Limit for Thyroglobulin Antibodies According to the National Academy of Clinical Biochemistry Guidelines: Comparison of Eleven Different Automated Methods. *Autoimmunity Highlights* 2017;8(1):8.

8. Rotmensch S, Cole LA. False Diagnosis and Needless Therapy of Presumed Malignant Disease in Women with False-Positive Human Chorionic Gonadotropin Concentrations. *Lancet* 2000;355(9205):712–5.

9. Hattori N, Ishihara T, Shimatsu A. Variability in the Detection of Macro TSH in Different Immunoassay Systems. *Eur J Endocrinol* 2016;174(1):9–15.

10. Rix M, Laurberg P, Porzig C, Kristensen SR. Elevated Thyroid-Stimulating Hormone Level in a Euthyroid Neonate Caused by Macro Thyrotropin-IgG Complex. *Acta Paediatrica* 2011;100(9):e135–7.

11. Bülow Pedersen I, Laurberg P. Biochemical Hyperthyroidism in a Newborn Baby Caused by Assay Interaction from Biotin Intake. *Eur Thyroid J* 2016;5(3):212–5.

12. Favresse J, Lardinois B, Nassogne MC, Preumont V, Maiter D, Gruson D. Anti-Streptavidin Antibodies Mimicking Heterophilic Antibodies in Thyroid Function Tests. *Clin Chem Lab Med* 2018;56(7):e160–e3.

13. Sakata S, Matsuda M, Ogawa T, Takuno H, Matsui I, Sarui H, Yasuda K. Prevalence of Thyroid Hormone Autoantibodies in Healthy Subjects. *Clin Endocrinol* 1994;41(3):365–70.

14. Lee M-N, Lee S-Y, Hur KY, Park H-D. Thyroxine (T4) Autoantibody Interference of Free T4 Concentration Measurement in a Patient With Hashimoto's Thyroiditis. *Ann Lab Med* 2017;37(2):169.

15. Lithwick-Yanai G, Dromi N, Shtabsky A, Morgenstern S, Strenov Y, Feinmesser M, et al. Multicentre Validation of a MicroRNA-Based Assay for Diagnosing Indeterminate Thyroid Nodules Utilising Fine Needle Aspirate Smears. *J Clin Pathol* 2017;70(6):500–7.

16. Pasquel FJ, Tsegka K, Wang H, Cardona S, Galindo RJ, Fayfman M, et al. Clinical Outcomes in Patients With Isolated or Combined Diabetic Ketoacidosis and Hyperosmolar Hyperglycemic State: A Retrospective, Hospital-Based Cohort Study. *Diabetes Care* 2020;43(2):349–57.
17. Loh TP, Kao SL, Halsall DJ, Toh S-AES, Chan E, Ho SC, et al. Macro-Thyrotropin: A Case Report and Review of Literature. *J Clin Endocrinol Metab* 2012;97(6):1823–8.
18. Francis GL, Waguespack SG, Bauer AJ, Angelos P, Benvenga S, Cerutti JM, et al. Management Guidelines for Children with Thyroid Nodules and Differentiated Thyroid Cancer. *Thyroid* 2015;25(7):716–59.
19. Mostoufi-Moab S, Labourier E, Sullivan L, LiVolsi V, Li Y, Xiao R, et al. Molecular Testing for Oncogenic Gene Alterations in Pediatric Thyroid Lesions. *Thyroid* 2018;28(1):60–7.
20. Ioachim, D. *The Bethesda System for Reporting Thyroid Cytopathology*. 2nd ed. Springer International Publishing; 2018. 236 p.
21. Patel KN, Angell TE, Babiarz J, Barth NM, Blevins T, Duh QY, et al. Performance of a Genomic Sequencing Classifier for the Preoperative Diagnosis of Cytologically Indeterminate Thyroid Nodules. *JAMA Surg* 2018;153(9):817–24.
22. Nikiforova MN, Mercurio S, Wald AI, Barbi de Moura M, Callenberg K, Santana-Santos L, et al. Analytical Performance of the ThyroSeq v3 Genomic Classifier for Cancer Diagnosis in Thyroid Nodules. *Cancer* 2018;124(8):1682–90.
23. Jackson S, Kumar G, Banizs AB, Toney N, Silverman JF, Narick CM, Finkelstein SD. Incremental Utility of Expanded Mutation Panel When Used in Combination with MicroRNA Classification in Indeterminate Thyroid Nodules. *Diagn Cytopathol* 2020;48(1):43–52.
24. Nishino M, Nikiforova M. Update on Molecular Testing for Cytologically Indeterminate Thyroid Nodules. *Arch Pathol Lab Med* 2018;142(4):446–57.

2

Imaging of the thyroid gland

PALLAVI IYER

INTRODUCTION

Given the location of the thyroid gland and biology of thyroid hormone synthesis, several different radiologic modalities maybe used, including scintigraphy, computed tomography, and ultrasound. The thyroid cell is comprised of follicular cells that under the direction thyrotropin can trap iodide (concentration gradient up to 20:1 to plasma) and incorporate it into thyroglobulin to produce thyroglobulin-bound thyroid hormones. This unique feature lends itself to being imaged using scintigraphy using iodide/iodide-like radiotracers (Figure 2.1). Given the location of the thyroid gland, it is easily imaged by a non-invasive method of ultrasonography. Further, CT scan and MRI with specific tracers that concentrate in metabolically active cells can be used to differentiate malignant vs. benign thyroid nodules (1). See Table 2.1 for comparison of the radiotracers used in thyroid imaging.

NIS-targeting radiopharmaceuticals

Technetium scan (Tc99m) pertechnetate ($^{99m}TcO_4^-$) is a radio-isotope that mimics iodine and is used for thyroid imaging. It is administered via intravenous

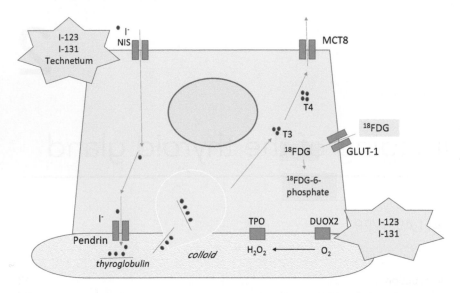

Figure 2.1 Depiction of a thyroid cell physiology and radiotracer activity.

injection and is trapped in the thyrocyte via the sodium iodide symporter in the thyroid cell. The thyroid gland is scanned 20 minutes after administration to reveal the location and size of the thyroid gland compared to the locations of the markers (Figure 2.2). This study is helpful in distinguishing between the causes of congenital hypothyroidism (sublingual thyroid gland, lingual thyroid gland, thyroid aplasia, and eutopic thyroid gland). Maternal blocking antibodies may sometimes interfere with the study and note an aplastic thyroid gland, but an ultrasound reveals a eutopic thyroid gland. This study is best performed when the TSH is elevated and thus upregulating the sodium-iodide symporter (NIS) expression (1, 2).

Radioactive uptake and scan

I-123 is a radiotracer with a half-life of 11 hours, making it ideal for diagnostic purposes. It is used to assess NIS-regulated function of the thyroid gland and iodide coupling and organification (DUOX2–TPO) needed for thyroid hormone synthesis. Defects in organification caused by dyshormonogenesis would result in the I-123 tracer being "washed out" easily by perchlorate discharge. The test involves administering I-123 and measuring uptake 2 hours post-administration. One hour later, an oral perchlorate is administered and another thyroid uptake image is obtained. With no organification defect, the perchlorate is unable to displace the I-123 that has been organified, but if the perchlorate rapidly displaces the I-123 (greater than 5–10% decrease in uptake), then a defect in an organification step is suspected.

Table 2.1 Comparison of radiotracers used in thyroid imaging

	I-123	Technetium	I-131	18FDG
Administration route	p.o.	i.v.	p.o.	i.v.
Half-life	13.2 hours	6.04 hours	8.06 days	110 min
Uses	Size and location of thyroid Uptake in focal masses uptake Detecting iodine organification defects (used with perchlorate discharge test) Differentiating etiology of hyperthyroidism Calculation of dose of I-131 for RAI for Graves' or differentiated thyroid cancer	Size and location of thyroid Uptake in focal masses uptake Lower cost	Ablate the thyroid gland Low dose for detection of thyroid tissue	Localize metabolically active disease
Limitations	Must be orally ingested Not readily available daily NIS needs to be upregulated (high TSH or thyroid-stimulating immunoglobulin)	Not organified—unable to assess organification defects	Long half-life	

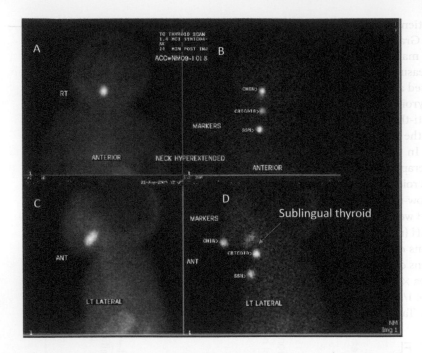

Figure 2.2 Patient with sublingual thyroid after $^{99m}TcO_4^-$ administration. A: anterior image after; B: anterior image of markers—chin, cricoid, and suprasternal notch (SSN), C: lateral image; D: markers superimposed with patient image.

I-123 uptake and scan is also useful in differentiating causes of hyperthyroidism (i.e., destructive thyroiditis, autonomously functioning nodule, Graves' disease, factitious thyrotoxicosis, or iodine overload). It can also help determine the ideal dose of therapeutic I-131 for the treatment of Graves' disease or the optimal dose for the treatment of papillary or follicular thyroid carcinoma. In Graves' disease, one would expect diffusely homogenous and increased uptake throughout the gland. In a destructive thyroiditis, the scan generally would illustrate low uptake diffusely. Alternatively, in an autonomously functioning nodule(s), increased focal uptake only in the area of the nodule (hot nodule) with concomitant suppressed uptake in the other areas would be noted (3). Of note, in adults, hot nodules are considered benign; however, in children, these nodules may still be of a malignant nature and surgical resection is recommended (4).

I-131 IMAGING AND THERAPY

Radioactive iodine is imported and trapped through the sodium-iodine symporter in the apical membrane of thyroid cell. The half-life of I-131 is 8 days; thus, it is mostly used for therapeutic purposes as it concentrates in thyrocytes and kills these cells over time. In low dose, I-131 may also be used for imaging in patients prior to ablation for post-thyroidectomy RAI therapy (similar to I-123). In Graves' disease, the goal of RAI therapy is to provide sufficient radiation dose to make the patient hypothyroid. The therapeutic dose (µCi) is calculated by measuring gland weight (g) × 50–200 µCi/g × (1/24 hour uptake in % administered activity) and generally estimates to ~15 mCi and renders the patient hypothyroid in about 1–2 months (3). The patient is prepared by discontinuing use of anti-thyroid medication for 5–7 days prior to the procedure to optimize uptake of the RAI (a low-iodine diet may also be used as adjuvant).

In patients with differentiated thyroid cancer (papillary and follicular), RAI therapy is indicated for ablating nodal, locoregional, and metastatic iodine-avid thyroid tissue that is not amenable to surgery. The patient is prepared by starting a low-iodine diet for 2 weeks and discontinuing thyroid hormone replacement for 2–3 weeks to achieve a TSH: >30 mIU/L or alternatively using recombinant human TSH (rhTSH) 0.9 mg intramuscularly given q24 hours for two doses to avoid symptoms of hypothyroidism prior to the procedure. Although more specific calculations could be made, an empiric dose based on the child's weight or body surface area × by dose typically used in adults may be use (e.g., 1.0–1.5 mCi/kg for 5 year old: 1/3 adult dose, 10 year old: 1/2 adult dose, and 15 year old: 5/6 of adult dose) (4). See Table 2.1 to compare the different radiotracers used in thyroid imaging.

18-FLURODEOXYGLUCOSE POSITRON EMISSION TOMOGRAPHY (^{18}FDG-PET) SCAN

^{18}FDG is used as a radiotracer to identify accelerated glucose metabolism due to upregulation of transmembrane glucose transporter (GLUT-1) in bioactive cells such as differentiated cancer cells. The introduced tracer in the cell is phosphorylated due to overexpression of hexokinases and traps the tracer in the form of ^{18}FDG-6-pohosphate (Figure 2.1). Thus, malignant thyroid cells that are metabolically active will concentrate this radiotracer (1). In patients with disseminated metastatic thyroid cancer, FDG-PET scan (along with post I-131 therapy scan) can help map the tumor burden. See Table 2.1 for a comparison of the different radiotracers used in thyroid imaging.

Thyroid ultrasound

Based on the anterior neck location, the thyroid gland can easily be viewed by a non-invasive method such as a thyroid ultrasound. Thyroid ultrasonography can detect and localize the thyroid gland and measure volume. With experienced ultrasonographers, an ultrasound could be employed to distinguish between different etiologies of congenital hypothyroidism—aplastic vs. eutopic vs. ectopic gland; however, ultrasonography could lead to a false result if hypoechoic structures near the trachea or thymic tissue are mistaken for thyroid tissue (2). If Doppler flow is also employed, an ultrasound can be helpful in distinguishing a hyper-functioning gland with increased blood flow from destructive thyroiditis with decreased blood flow (3).

The best use of thyroid ultrasound is to define thyroid nodules. If on physical exam, a thyroid nodule is palpated or a thyroid nodule is found incidentally on another imaging study, a thyroid ultrasound is recommended for further characterization of the nodule. There are certain ultrasonographic characteristics that suggest higher risk of malignancy that warrant fine needle aspiration (FNA) to review cytopathology. In children being evaluated for thyroid nodules, characteristics such as size of at least 1 cm of solid composition, hypoechogenicity, irregular margins, increased blood flow to the nodule, microcalcifications, and associated abnormal-appearing cervical lymph nodes are most concerning and should be considered for fine needle aspiration (4). Children with autoimmune thyroiditis who have asymmetric thyroid enlargement or palpable cervical lymph nodes should also have a thyroid ultrasound performed looking for microcalcification to detect infiltrative papillary thyroid carcinoma (4). The American Thyroid Association (ATA) management guidelines suggest that suspicious patterns can help stratify risk of thyroid malignancy and decisions to proceed with FNA based on the size of the lesion. Suspicious characteristics defined here include the presence of microcalcifications, hypoechogenicity of the nodule, irregular margins, taller than wide on transverse view; however, intranodular blood flow was not indicative of malignancy especially papillary thyroid carcinoma (5). In adults, the size of the nodule along with its characteristics helps in the decision of whether to proceed with an FNA. For the most suspicious pattern, size threshold of 1 cm is warranted, low suspicion pattern—1.5 cm, and for a very low suspicion lesion—threshold of 2 cm nodule is used (5). Another thyroid ultrasound reporting system is the American College of Radiology thyroid imaging, reporting, and data system (ACR-TI-RADS) that uses total point determination to stratify risk of differentiated thyroid cancer with TR 1 (benign) to TR 5 (highly suspicious). Based on the results of the risk stratification and size of the nodule, ACR-TI-RADS results guide the need and interval for ultrasound follow-up vs. fine needle aspiration (FNA)(6). Both the ATA and the ACR TI-RADS have been validated in children with few caveats including sclerosing variant papillary thyroid carcinoma presenting with diffuse infiltration full of punctate lesions (without necessarily a focal lesion), presence of intrathyroid thymic rest tissue, higher prevalence of metastases to the lymph nodes, and higher prevalence of malignancy in intermediate nodules (7). Although both ATA and ACR TI-RADS system are helpful in determining risk of cancer and thus the need for FNA, the size threshold has not been validated in children.

COMPUTED TOMOGRAPHY (CT) AND MAGNETIC RESONANCE IMAGING

Generally, CT and MRI are not required for characterization of the thyroid gland. However, CT of the neck and lung can be helpful to characterize cervical and mediastinal lymph nodes along with lung parenchyma in patients with thyroid cancer (papillary and medullary). For soft tissue extension such as in bone marrow, liver, and abdominal lymph nodes, MRI is used (8). These modalities are especially used when planning a re-operation for metastatic thyroid cancer or for prognosis and planning for chemotherapy.

REFERENCES

1. Giovanella L, Avram AM, Iakovou I, Kwak J, Lawson SA, Lulaj E, et al. EANM Practice Guideline/SNMMI Procedure Standard for RAIU and Thyroid Scintigraphy. *Eur J Nucl Med Mol Imaging* 2019;46(12):2514–25.
2. Livett T, LaFranchi S. Imaging in Congenital Hypothyroidism. *Curr Opin Pediatr* 2019;31(4):555–61.
3. Ross DS, Burch HB, Cooper DS, Greenlee MC, Laurberg P, Maia AL, et al. 2016 American Thyroid Association Guidelines for Diagnosis and Management of Hyperthyroidism and Other Causes of Thyrotoxicosis. *Thyroid* 2016;26(10):1343–421.
4. Francis GL, Waguespack SG, Bauer AJ, Angelos P, Benvenga S, Cerutti JM, et al. Management Guidelines for Children with Thyroid Nodules and Differentiated Thyroid Cancer. *Thyroid* 2015;25(7):716–59.
5. Haugen BR, Alexander EK, Bible KC, Doherty GM, Mandel SJ, Nikiforov YE, et al. 2015 American Thyroid Association Management Guidelines for Adult Patients with Thyroid Nodules and Differentiated Thyroid Cancer: The American Thyroid Association Guidelines Task Force on Thyroid Nodules and Differentiated Thyroid Cancer. *Thyroid* 2016;26(1):1–133.
6. Tessler FN, Middleton WD, Grant EG, Hoang JK, Berland LL, Teefey SA, et al. ACR Thyroid Imaging, Reporting and Data System (TI-RADS): White Paper of the ACR TI-RADS Committee. *J Am Coll Radiol* 2017;14(5):587–95.
7. Martinez-Rios C, Daneman A, Bajno L, van der Kaay DCM, Moineddin R, Wasserman JD. Utility of Adult-Based Ultrasound Malignancy Risk Stratifications in Pediatric Thyroid Nodules. *Pediatr Radiol* 2018;48(1):74–84.
8. Kushchayev SV, Kushchayeva YS, Tella SH, Glushko T, Pacak K, Teytelboym OM. Medullary Thyroid Carcinoma: An Update on Imaging. *J Thyroid Res* 2019;2019:1893047.

Congenital hypothyroidism

GAIL MICK

SUMMARY

Thyroid hormone is essential for normal development, especially during the first several years of life when crucial brain and somatic growth are in progress. Since its inception in developed countries during the 1970s, newborn screening (NBS) for congenital hypothyroidism (CH) has essentially eradicated the neurocognitive disability of this condition. Over the past several decades, earlier diagnosis as well as treatment with higher doses of levothyroxine has further improved outcomes. Regrettably, despite its proven lifetime impact, estimates indicate that only 30% of the 127 million babies born annually worldwide are screened for CH. The disorders of CH include a wide array of primary hypothyroidism (PH) due to developmental/genetic defects in the thyroid gland as well as central hypothyroidism (CCH) due to aberrant hypothalamic-pituitary regulation of the thyroid. An understanding of the pathophysiology of CH, as well as guidelines and challenges in NBS, is essential for best practice diagnosis and management. As NBS protocols and diagnostic cut-offs have improved, the prevalence of CH has increased due to the detection of milder cases. Adding to this, premature infants have spawned an upsurge in transient and permanent CH related to hypothalamic–pituitary–thyroid axis immaturity and complex medical care. Further research and understanding are needed regarding the risks and benefits of treating these milder cases of CH. Nevertheless, current management requires rapid diagnosis of affected infants and treatment ideally by 2 weeks of age with 10–15 microgram/kg/day of levothyroxine. Frequent follow-up visits to evaluate growth, development, and thyroid levels are also essential to maintain optimal outcomes. Properly managed, patients with CH have an excellent long-term prognosis.

INTRODUCTION

Congenital hypothyroidism (CH) encompasses disorders of the thyroid gland (primary hypothyroidism [PH]) and pituitary/hypothalamic axis (central hypothyroidism [CCH]). Rare disorders in peripheral thyroid hormone transport and action are also included but not discussed herein. CH is further categorized as permanent (lifelong thyroid hormone requirement) and transient (temporary hypothyroidism identified at birth that resolves by 2–3 years of age). The latter group often includes premature infants and those with milder forms of CH associated with eutopic (normal size and positioned) thyroid glands.

CH is the most common cause of preventable intellectual disability, yet approximately 70% of babies worldwide do not undergo newborn screening (NBS) for CH. Globally, maternal iodine-deficient hypothyroidism is especially consequential because the fetus relies entirely on maternal thyroid hormone production prior to developing its own functioning thyroid tissue at 10–12 weeks gestation. Universal salt iodination is the strategy to eliminate this nutritional deficiency. Despite hypothyroidism, most babies with CH appear normal at birth. Two factors are protective to the fetal brain, (1) maternal thyroid production provides 25–50% of the fetal requirement, and (2) enhanced intracerebral conversion of T4 to its biologically active metabolite T3, maximizes hormone efficacy. Hence, for CH infants of mothers with normal thyroid function, neurocognitive outcomes are excellent when there is early detection by NBS and prompt treatment (1).

PRIMARY CH

Thyroid dysplasia (TD) compromises 85% of cases of PH and includes complete agenesis (15–33% by scintigraphy), hemi-agenesis, hypoplasia, and ectopy (48–51% of TD by scintigraphy). Ectopy results from incomplete caudal migration of the primordial thyroid anlage from its locus near the base of the tongue to its final position anterior to the trachea. Ectopic remnant tissue is dysplastic and insufficient for postnatal thyroid hormone requirements. Genetic causes for TD are rarely identified but can include transcription factor mutations in the development of the thyroid gland and other tissues. Five monogenic causes of TD (with either autosomal dominant [AD] or recessive [AR] inheritance) are worth noting, (1) TSH receptor inactivating mutations, including G-protein signaling defects (AR), (2) NXK2-1 or brain-lung thyroid syndrome (AD), (3) PAX8 (AD), (4) FOXE-1 or Bamforth–Lazarus syndrome (AR), and (5) NKX2-5.

Genetic causes of thyroid hormone biosynthesis (dyshormonogenesis) encompass roughly 10–15% of PH and are usually AR/homozygous at presentation. Mild heterozygous variants can cause hypothyroidism that may or may not be detected by NBS. The thyroid hormone biosynthetic process requires several sequential steps that, if lacking, may cause PH. First, iodide in the blood accumulates in the thyroid cell via the basal membrane *sodium/iodide symporter* (NIS) and, subsequently, by the apical membrane pendrin complex (SLC26A4/PDS). *Thyroid peroxidase* (TPO) catalyzed the iodination of tyrosine residues on thyroglobulin (TG) as well as the coupling of these iodinated tyrosines to form 3,5,5'-triiodothyronine (T3) and 3,5,3'5', tetraiodothyronine (T4). The organification process of TPO requires hydrogen peroxide produced by *dual oxidase 1* (DUOX1) and *dual oxidase 2* (DUOX2). The *iodotyrosine dehalogenase 1* (DEHAL1) rescues and recycles iodotyrosines that are not incorporated into free thyroid hormone. A palpable goiter and familial history of CH are often present with disorders of thyroid hormone biosynthesis.

Clinical clues that suggest syndromic causes of CH include hearing loss (Pendred's syndrome, SLC26A4/PDS), cleft palate (Bamforth–Lazarus syndrome, FOXE1), urogenital malformations (PAX-8), cardiac malformations (NKX2-5), infantile respiratory distress disorder and chorea (NK2X-1), and DiGeorge syndrome with cardiac malformation (TBX1). Consumptive hypothyroidism due to excess type 3 deiodinase (hepatic hemangiomas) or protein loss (congenital nephrotic syndrome) can lead to treatment-worthy neonatal primary hypothyroidism pending resolution of the underlying etiology.

With improvements in CH detection protocols, roughly 30–40% of CH babies present with eutopic thyroid glands (normal position and size). Eutopic CH is often transient but may also be permanent wherein mild defects in thyroid hormone synthesis are presumed. Maternal factors including iodine deficiency or excess, as well as trans-placental acquired maternal TSH-receptor blocking antibodies may cause varying degrees of eutopic hypothyroxinemia in the newborn. Transient eutopic primary CH is also a frequent diagnosis in premature and critically ill neonates. Postnatal factors such as excess iodine exposure from topical antiseptics and radiographic contrast agents may cause hypothyroxinemia. These infants are often committed to a 3-year course of levothyroxine before the final diagnosis (transient or permanent CH) is elucidated by a short trial off levothyroxine.

CENTRAL CH

The prevalence of central congenital hypothyroidism (CCH) is broadly reported at between 1:16,000 and 1:100,000. It may be detected by NBS if primary T4-based methods are employed; however many cases are diagnosed during infancy and childhood. Clinical clues that may be associated with CCH include midline defects (cleft lip/palate, hypertelorism, nystagmus) as well as evidence for other pituitary hormone deficiencies. Cholestatic hepatitis with jaundice is a recognized neonatal presentation of panhypopituitarism with CCH. Associated central adrenal insufficiency and growth hormone deficiency may present with hypoglycemia, poor feeding, and cardiovascular compromise. Of importance concerning the treatment of CCH with combined hypopituitarism, recommendations support identifying and treating any associated central adrenal insufficiency prior to commencing thyroid hormone in order to avoid precipitating latent adrenal crisis. Genetic defects in pituitary/hypothalamic development, brain tumors, and isolated deficiency of TRH/TSH production may also present as CCH. Rare mutations in the TSH beta-subunit may cause impaired TSH signaling and a perplexing picture of low to high TSH values related to laboratory methodology. Transient causes of CCH often present in the context of acute perinatal illness and include euthyroid sick syndrome and exposure to agents that suppress pituitary hypothalamic function such as glucocorticoids and dopamine.

NEWBORN SCREENING

Early detection and treatment of CH by newborn screening (NBS) avert the classic clinical phenotype of CH and its serious neurodevelopmental sequelae. In developed countries, the prevalence of CH has increased over the past several decades from 1:3500 births to roughly 1:1800. Factors responsible for this trend include improved (lower) NBS diagnostic cut-off values, demographic shifts, and increased numbers of very premature infants. Overall, there is a higher incidence of CH in Hispanics and Asians, with multiple births and prematurity. NBS methods vary concerning whether T4, TSH, both T4 and TSH, or primary T4 with reflex TSH is measured on the neonatal bloodspot specimen (2). Each approach has advantages with primary TSH being the most sensitive method. Combination T4/TSH methods may detect CCH and thyroid-binding globulin (TBG) deficiency. To convert the whole blood, filter card screen TSH value (mU/L) to a comparable serum TSH, multiply by 2.2. For example, a bloodspot TSH = 20 mU/L equates to a serum TSH = 44 mU/L. During the first 24 hours of life, a physiologic surge in TSH negates the diagnostic value of this transitional interval. In the US, the initial NBS specimen is obtained prior to hospital discharge (at 24–72 hours of age). This early discharge timing necessitates a higher initial bloodspot TSH cut-off to avoid excessive false positive results related to the residual post-natal TSH surge. By 2–4 weeks of age, normal infants have a serum TSH <10 mU/L. Some states perform a second bloodspot sample at 1–6 weeks of age that detects up to 20% more cases, including permanent CH (3). The severity of CH is defined according to serum free T4 at diagnosis and ranges from severe (free T4 <0.39 ng/dL) to mild (free T4 = 0.78–1.16 ng/dL). Preterm and acutely ill infants should have serial follow-up NBS to detect gestational age-related trends in thyroid function as well as deviations related to critical illness. In particular, iodinated contrast agents, dopamine, and glucocorticoids adversely affect neonatal thyroid levels.

CLINICAL PRESENTATION

The classic clinical findings of severe, untreated CH are uncommon due to early detection but can include prolonged jaundice, cold and mottled skin, large tongue, umbilical hernia, facial puffiness, and open posterior fontanelle. Additional features are lethargy, poor feeding, constipation, and post-term gestation. The presence of a goiter suggests a defect in thyroid hormone synthesis. It is important to consider other potentially associated conditions including congenital heart disease, hearing loss, Trisomy 21, and genetic or syndromic thyroid disorders (discussed in the Primary CH section). Medical history should consider excess iodine exposure, maternal thyroid disease, and siblings with CH.

CONFIRMATORY THYROID TESTING

NBS blood spot test results can be interpreted and triaged based on "ACT" sheets and algorithms provided by the American College of Medical Genetics (ACMG) (www.acmg.net/ACMG/Medical-Genetics-Practice-Resources/ACT_Sheets_ and_Algorithms.aspx). State health departments also prepare region-specific NBS result guidelines on their websites. Consensus statements recommend that if the initial bloodspot TSH ≥40 (at >24 hours of age), treatment with levothyroxine should commence pending confirmatory serum thyroid testing (free T4 and TSH). If the bloodspot TSH <40, then repeat bloodspot or serum labs can be resulted prior to beginning treatment. Persistent elevations of serum TSH >20 should be treated even if free T4 is normal. A baseline thyroglobulin is also helpful as an index of residual thyroid tissue and complements diagnostic imaging interpretation. If maternal autoimmune thyroiditis is present, infant or maternal testing should include TSH receptor blocking antibodies. If excess iodine exposure is suspected in either the newborn or nursing mother, measuring urinary iodine may be helpful. Thyroid-binding globulin (TBG) levels should be determined if X-linked TBG deficiency is suggested by bloodspot results demonstrating low T4 and normal TSH in an otherwise healthy male infant. If central hypothyroidism is a concern, pituitary/hypothalamic initial testing should include electrolytes, glucose, cortisol, and growth hormone testing.

DIAGNOSTIC IMAGING

Initial imaging in newborns with CH. The initial diagnostic thyroid imaging method aims to localize and quantify thyroid tissue. This anatomical information is especially helpful when counseling parents concerning the long-term medical plan. Color Doppler ultrasound (US) delineates thyroid volume and whether it is normal, enlarged, or hypoplastic. In an active newborn, however, it is possible to miss small amounts of ectopic thyroid tissue. Serum thyroglobulin, which reflects thyroid tissue content, is a helpful complementary study in this situation. If thyroid tissue is not identified on US but blood TG is detectable, then ectopic tissue is likely. If the thyroid gland is large but TG is undetectable, then a homozygous TG mutation is certain. Technetium 99m (Tc99m) scintigraphy is the easiest method for identifying *functioning* thyroid tissue because the isotope enters by the thyrocyte sodium-iodide symporter (NIS). A disadvantage, however, is that the test relies on an elevated TSH for Tc99m uptake and, hence, it must be obtained before or during the first week of levothyroxine therapy. For families who travel long distances for medical care, this option may not be achievable. Iodine[123] scintigraphy is analogous to Tc99m outside of the incorporation of iodine[123] into endogenous thyroxine. It is not practical for newborn imaging because the isotope must be preordered and the test duration is longer. Bilateral knee radiographs should be obtained in cases of severe CH to evaluate bone maturation. An absence of the normal femoral and tibial epiphyseal nuclei correlates with a poorer neurocognitive outcome.

Later diagnostic imaging. After 3 years of age, when the potential neurocognitive harm of brief hypothyroxinemia is deemed negligible, thyroid treatment may be tapered or discontinued to conduct Tc99m imaging. Repeating the initial ultrasound can also shed light on previously borderline anatomy. If dyshormonogenesis is suspected, iodine[123] uptake with perchlorate discharge will identify defects in iodine uptake and organification.

PRETERM INFANTS

Preterm infants account for 10–17% of babies with CH, despite representing roughly 1% of the newborns screened. Those babies with extreme low birth weight (<1000 g) or very low birth weight (1000–1500 g) present unique challenges regarding the detection and treatment of CH. Prematurity leads to a delay in the normal postnatal TSH surge (dTSH), with associated hypothyroxinemia, that is attributed to transitional immaturity of the pituitary hypothalamic axis. Retrospective cohort studies indicate that the dTSH occurs at between 2 and 8 weeks of age and with an incidence as high as 1:64 infants born at <32 weeks of age. Because of the high prevalence of dTSH in premature infants, recommendations suggest that these babies have 2–3 serial NBS or serum free T4 and TSH measurements between birth and 16 weeks of life (depending on gestational age). The limited, longitudinal follow-up studies of premature infants with dTSH reveal a spectrum of final diagnoses, including transient CH, and persistent mild hyperthyrotropinemia (mild TSH elevation with normal free T4) as well as some permanent CH. Whether infants with dTSH suffer adverse long-term neurocognitive consequences from mild or transient CH is unresolved.

TREATMENT

Once confirmatory serum labs are obtained on a newborn with suspected CH, treatment should begin promptly with 10–15 mcg/kg/day of oral levothyroxine pending lab results. The highest dose range is recommended for infants with severe hypothyroxinemia. Tablets of levothyroxine are crushed and administered to the infant in a small volume of water or milk. Where feasible, families should be instructed to avoid simultaneous administration of soy formula, antireflux medications, oral calcium, and iron supplements because they impair the gastric absorption of levothyroxine.

FOLLOW-UP

After commencing treatment, an initial lab test at 1–2 weeks aims to achieve normalization of thyroid hormone levels. Thereafter, it is beneficial to measure serum free T4 and TSH every month until age 6 months, every 1–2 months until age 12 months, and then every 3–4 months until age 3 years. After age 3 years, twice-yearly thyroid testing is usually adequate. Patients with complete thyroid agenesis or those in whom medication compliance is suboptimal may require more frequent testing. The goal of treatment is to maintain the serum free T4 in the upper range of normal and TSH between 2 and 4 mU/L. Longitudinal data have affirmed that prompt normalization of hypothyroxinemia maximizes cognitive outcomes. On the other hand, over-treatment, which is defined as persistent supernormal elevations of serum T4 with suppressed TSH, also has adverse neurocognitive consequences. Regular clinical follow-up should include careful review of growth and developmental progress. If neurocognitive or language delay are detected, early referrals for developmental intervention services are essential.

REEVALUATION

For patients with normal thyroid gland anatomy, a trial off levothyroxine is considered at 3 years of age. Patients who have maintained all TSH values less than 10 mU/L on treatment (after 1 year of age), and who required minimal to absent dose increases since birth, are more likely to successfully discontinue levothyroxine. If all serum TSH remain <6 mU/L with normal free T4 after discontinuing levothyroxine, the diagnosis of transient CH is confirmed. If TSH remains between 6 and <10 with normal free T4, serial laboratory follow-up is recommended to evaluate for concerning trends. An increase in TSH ≥10 and/or a progressive decrease in free T4 is abnormal and supports restarting levothyroxine. The long-term outcome of patients with persistent mild hyperthyrotropinemia (TSH 6–8) with normal free T4 is controversial. Potential etiologies for this pattern of thyroid labs include minor TSH receptor mutations that alter TSH binding or post receptor (G-protein) signaling. Case series indicate that about 54%

of CH patients with eutopic glands are found to have transient CH and come off treatment. Patients with Trisomy 21 have a lifetime risk for thyroid dysregulation, making a trial off therapy less desirable.

LONG-TERM OUTCOME

The profound intellectual disability (IQ <70) associated with untreated CH prior to the advent of NBS has essentially vanished. Yet, longitudinal follow-up of some treated patients continues to reveal minor neurocognitive and behavioral deficits that correlate with initial age of treatment and the severity of birth hypothyroxinemia. Parsing out confounding variables such a socio-educational status and the longitudinal adequacy of thyroid replacement therapy remains problematic. Yet, the overall prognosis for early-treated patients remains both excellent and noteworthy for unfettered educational achievement with normal societal integration.

REFERENCES

1. Leger J, Olivieri A, Donaldson M, Torresani T, Krude H, van Vliet G, et al. European Society for Paediatric Endocrinology Consensus Guidelines on Screening, Diagnosis, and Management of Congenital Hypothyroidism. *J Clin Endocrinol Metab* 2014;99(2):363–84.
2. LaFranchi SH. Approach to the Diagnosis and Treatment of Neonatal Hypothyroidism. *J Clin Endocrinol Metab* 2011;96(10):2959–67.
3. Connelly KJ, Lafranchi SH. Detection of Neonates with Mild Congenital Hypothyroidism (Primary) or Isolated Hyperthyrotropinemia: An Increasingly Common Management Dilemma. *Expert Rev Endocrinol Metab* 2014;9(3):263–71.

4

Acquired hypothyroidism

GRACE DOUGAN AND ANNE LENZ

Acquired hypothyroidism in the developed world is primarily caused by auto-immune thyroid disease (AITD). It is the leading cause of thyroid disorders in the pediatric population in the US (1). In the underdeveloped world, iodine deficiency, or endemic goiter, remains an important cause of hypothyroidism, affecting one-third of the world's population (2). Less common causes of acquired primary hypothyroidism include subacute thyroiditis, acute iodine toxicity, postoperative hypothyroidism, radiation exposure, chromosomal abnormalities, and medication-related hypothyroidism. Secondary and tertiary acquired causes of hypothyroidism are less common and directly related to pituitary and hypothalamic insults (tumor, hypo perfusion, hypophysitis, local radiation, postoperative and brain trauma).

AUTOIMMUNE THYROID DISEASE

In 1912, Dr. Hakaru Hashimoto first described a series of four female patients with the distinct presence of inflammatory cells, local fibrosis, and loss of typical thyroid cell architecture not seen in already established pathologies of the time. This was later recognized as an independent disorder and is now commonly known as Hashimoto's disease or autoimmune thyroiditis. Autoimmune thyroiditis is caused by a T-cell mediated infiltration of the thyroid gland and presents with a spectrum of disease from incidental goiter, to subclinical hypothyroidism, to overt thyroid dysfunction. The onset of hypothyroid symptoms can be slow in progression, and the majority of patients will be biochemically and clinically euthyroid at diagnosis. Symptoms tend to be nonspecific and overlapping of other disorders. Patients tend to complain of low energy, depression, cold intolerance, thinning hair, dry skin, rash, mild weight gain, constipation, short stature, pubertal delay in the adolescent patient, and menstrual irregularity. Physical exam findings vary from an isolated non-tender goiter to carotenemia, bradycardia, slowing of the return-phase of deep tendon reflexes, thelarche in the absence of pubarche, linear growth plateau, and myxedema. The goiter associated with AITD is generally symmetric and firm or rubbery on palpation with an irregular or pebbly capsule and painless. Thyroid nodules may occur with increased frequency in AITD and should be monitored in the same fashion as thyroid nodules attributable to other causes (3). The sequelae of severe, prolonged untreated hypothyroidism can include anemia, elevated total and LDL cholesterol, elevated creatinine and liver enzymes, and pseudo menarche. Skeletal maturation slows in overt hypothyroidism and bone age is often delayed, sometimes coinciding with the onset of disease but discordant with the pubertal exam (Figure 4.1). Select cases of severe hypothyroidism have identified pituitary and sella turcica enlargement due to hyperplasia of thyrotropes producing TSH. In a small number of cases, AITD may present with a brief period of mild hyperthyroidism related to the release of pre-formed thyroid hormone within the gland called "Hashitoxicosis." Following this transient period of thyroid hormone excess, hypothyroidism ensues. There remains a significant percentage of adolescents who will achieve complete remission of mild thyroid hypo function over time, and treatment may not be indicated if labs are consistent with subclinical hypothyroidism.

Once euthyroid, symptoms and sequelae attributed to hypothyroidism should resolve, though goiter may persist even with adequate thyroid hormone replacement (Figure 4.2). Skin and hair findings may take longer to completely resolve owing to the time necessary for renewal of new hair and skin cells, including initial increased loss of hair followed by resumption of the normal hair cycle. Other causes of fatigue, depression, constipation, and accompanying symptoms should be pursued when thyroid function testing is normal or only mildly abnormal.

Obesity itself can cause a mild elevation of TSH (usually TSH <8 mIU/mL) called hyperthyrotropinemia of obesity and should be differentiated from intrinsic thyroid pathology or AITD. Screening patients for hypothyroidism in the setting of isolated significant obesity and non-specific symptoms of fatigue or depression can frequently yield mildly abnormal results. Symptoms in children with these clinical complaints should not be solely attributed to thyroid disease nor would symptoms be expected to improve with the treatment of mildly elevated TSH levels and normal free thyroxine levels. Significant weight reduction through diet and exercise will normalize thyroid function labs in hyperthyrotropinemia of obesity (4, 5). Current medical evidence does not identify a medical advantage in treatment or support treating obese children with subclinical hypothyroidism.

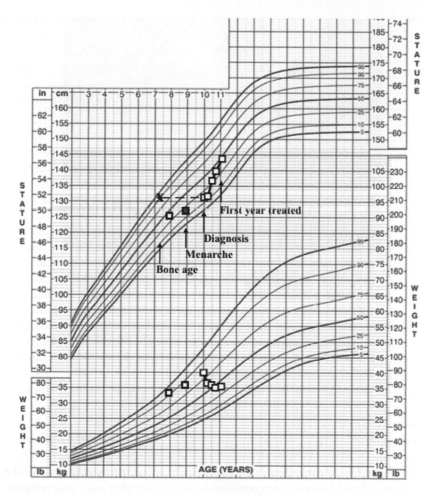

Figure 4.1 A 10-year-old previously healthy female presents with the primary complaint of short stature on her routine well child exam. Bone age (X) was delayed 3.5 years, but the child was menarchal at 9 years of age and breasts were Tanner 4 on the initial exam with the absence of pubic hair. TSH was found to be profoundly elevated and with the initiation of levothyroxine, linear growth accelerated, weight became proportional, and breast tissue regressed with the absence of menses in the first year of treatment. This is a rare example of Van Wyk–Grumbach syndrome.

OTHER CAUSES OF ACQUIRED PRIMARY HYPOTHYROIDISM

Subacute thyroiditis presents with a tender, enlarged thyroid gland, likely due to viral mediated inflammation. Fever may be present along with other viral symptoms initially. Hyperthyroidism or hypothyroidism may be associated with

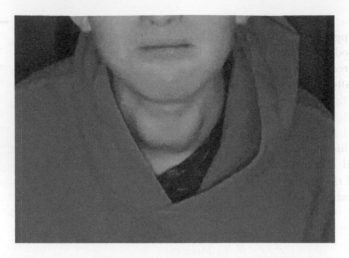

Figure 4.2 A 10-year-old child with autoimmune thyroid disease, biochemically euthyroid with remaining moderate goiter.

subacute thyroiditis and typically lasts for 1–2 months. NSAIDS or corticosteroids may improve tenderness of the gland and beta-blockers can ameliorate symptoms of hyperthyroidism. Hypothyroidism is treated with levothyroxine as with AITD, but may be transient and short-lived.

Both iodine deficiency and excess can result in hypothyroidism. Primary sources of dietary iodine include iodized salt, seaweed, kelp, iodine-containing bread and dough conditioners, eggs, and dairy products. Iodine-containing supplements and vitamins are also an important source of iodine intake. The normal recommended intake of iodine from dietary and supplemental sources is 150 ug/day in adults. Low-iodine diets causing deficiency typically are <50 ug/day. The American Thyroid Association recommends that any supplemental iodine intake should be <500 ug/day to avoid toxic effects of excess iodine. Exposure to excess iodine can also come from iodine-containing contrast agents for radiological studies, cardiac catheterizations, or iodine-containing topical preparations such as betadine. Infants and premature babies are at higher risk for iodine exposure through surgical preparation using betadine given their small surface area and skin maturity. Exposure to excess iodine induces the Wolff–Chaikoff effect, reducing thyroid hormone production by inhibition of thyroid iodide organification. Most individuals will escape this reduction of thyroid hormone production in 7–10 days, but other individuals demonstrate prolonged hypothyroidism after exposure to excess iodine. Patients with previous thyroid pathology (thyroid surgery, subacute thyroiditis, AITD, etc.) and neonates seem to have a higher propensity towards prolonged hypothyroidism after large iodine exposure. Transient congenital hypothyroidism in babies born to women taking excessive iodine during pregnancy and lactation has been reported (6, 7). Serum iodine levels are not reliable markers of iodine sufficiency due to daily variation; however, urinary iodine levels >300 µg/L are considered excessive in children and adults with levels >500 µg/L considered excessive in pregnant women. Thyroglobulin levels in dried blood spots may also be an indicator of iodine status (8).

Acquired hypothyroidism related to iatrogenic causes includes hypothyroidism after complete thyroidectomy or hemithyroidectomy for either thyroid nodules, thyroid cancer, or Graves' disease. Hypothyroidism after radioactive iodine ablation of hyperthyroidism is the goal of ablation (9). Patients should be counseled in these clinical situations that thyroid hormone replacement will be required lifelong.

Several chromosomal abnormalities are known to be associated with an increased risk for hypothyroidism including Downs syndrome and Turner syndrome and to a lesser degree Klinefelter's syndrome. Ten to 30% of girls with Turner syndrome develop AITD, and screening of thyroid function should occur at diagnosis and then every 1–2 years thereafter (10). Thyroid disease is also more common in Downsyndrome and is attributable to AITD, congenital hypothyroidism, and mild dyshormonogenesis. Screening for thyroid disease in trisomy 21 should occur at 6 and 12 months of life and annually thereafter (11). If TSH becomes elevated, therapy with levothyroxine should be initiated and dose titrated as with AITD. In Klinefelter's syndrome, autoimmunity tends to have a higher incidence in the adult patient. Evidence does not support the routine evaluation of thyroid function in the pediatric KS patient, but studies support annual screening by age 10 or sooner for symptoms of thyroid disease (12).

Several medications are known to induce hypothyroidism via inhibition of thyroid hormone secretion (lithium, amiodarone, aminoglutethimide), via thyroiditis (interferon, interleukin-2, sunitinib), or via TSH suppression (glucocorticoids, dopamine agonists, somatostatin analogues, rexinoids, carbamazepine, oxcarbazepine) (13). Hypothyroidism generally remits after the discontinuation of these medications, and the treatment of drug-induced hypothyroidism is no different than the treatment of autoimmune hypothyroidism.

DIAGNOSTIC EVALUATION

Once the clinical history and exam bring into question the function of the thyroid gland, laboratory studies should be pursued first. The recommended primary evaluation for acquired primary hypothyroidism is the measurement of a serum TSH. There are current recommendations against the routine screening of thyroid function in the obese child with a reassuring linear growth pattern in the absence of goiter or early puberty (14). The third-generation TSH assays have a functional sensitivity below 0.020 mIU/L and are replacing the previous second-generation assays. In primary hypothyroidism, TSH will be elevated. Free thyroxine (FT4) levels would be the next recommended value to be measured if the TSH is abnormal. FT4 will be normal in subclinical disease, but levels will become low as the severity of thyroid disease increases. Free thyroid index (FTI) is a product of the total thyroxine and triiodothyronine uptake (T3U). With primary hypothyroidism the FTI is a marker of low serum free thyroxine. Direct measurement of FT4 has replaced the need to calculate the FTI in settings of abnormal serum thyroid binding proteins. Elevated thyroid peroxidase antibodies and antithyroglobulin antibodies can confirm AITD as the underlying etiology of hypothyroidism. A small subset of patients with AITD will have negative thyroid autoantibodies despite pathologic evidence of lymphocytic infiltration of the gland. A study suggests that the disease process may be milder in antibody-negative thyroiditis (15). Free T4 value by equilibrium dialysis assay is an additional option when confounding factors suggest the standard FT4 may not match the clinical picture or TSH result. Biotin is a known substance that interferes with lab assays for FT4. The cessation of this vitamin for 72 hours prior is suggested by most labs to improve the reliability of the results. T3 and reverse T3 levels have no purpose in the evaluation of acquired hypothyroidism and should not be used alone as a laboratory determinant of thyroid disease in the outpatient setting.

In secondary and tertiary acquired hypothyroidism, the preferred screening evaluation is a direct measurement of free thyroxine as well as the TSH. TSH alone is a less reliable assay for screening, as results can vary between low, normal, and elevated values. Isolated thyroid deficiency is rare in secondary/tertiary hypothyroidism and additional pituitary deficiency should be screened as well.

Ultrasound of the thyroid gland is not required in most cases of hypothyroidism. However, ultrasound may be indicated in the following clinical scenarios: physical exam of the thyroid gland is limited by a larger pre-cervical fat pad; goiter is large enough to prohibit a reliable exam for nodule; asymmetric goiter; or discrete palpable nodule is identifiable.

TREATMENT OF ACQUIRED PRIMARY HYPOTHYROIDISM

Treatment of acquired primary hypothyroidism may include observation in cases of subclinical disease, typically when the TSH <10 mIU/mL. Laboratory evaluation is recommended every 6–12 months, taking into consideration the rate of spontaneous remission in as many as 30% of adolescent patients (16). In cases of overt hypothyroidism or TSH >10 mIU/mL, thyroid hormone replacement with levothyroxine is indicated as the standard of care (17). Depending on the degree of hypothyroidism, the initial dose may need to be reduced and increased to a therapeutic level over days to weeks. Common symptoms of overtreatment or intolerance of thyroid hormone replacement include sleep difficulties, academic decline, myopathies, or headache. The headache is secondary to transient increased intracranial hypertension from the increased production of cerebral spinal fluid ahead of the ability to drain the intracranial spaces. Dose reduction until symptoms remit and reattempts at increasing the dose over a few weeks result in improved tolerance. As levothyroxine increases serum T4 levels, an endogenous dose adjustment occurs as deiodinases allow for the conversion of T4 to bioactive T3 according to the body's needs. Levothyroxine doses for complete thyroid hormone replacement are higher in younger children than pubertal and adult patients. Typical full replacement doses expressed as mcg/kg/day are as follows: infants 10–15, toddlers and preschoolers 6–10; pre-pubertal to early pubertal children 2–4; and adults 1.5–2. Lower doses may be sufficient depending on the degree of TSH elevation. Levothyroxine can help control goiter in some patients and has been used in the euthyroid or subclinical patient with AITD and goiter (18). Due to the long half-life of levothyroxine (7 days), repeat thyroid function testing with TSH and free T4 levels should be completed 6 weeks after the initiation of therapy and after all dose changes, with the goal of keeping thyroid hormone levels in the middle of the normal range. Testing in growing children should be repeated every 4–6 months; once linear growth is complete, testing may be spaced to every 6–12 months. Ideally, levothyroxine is given on an empty stomach, but the risk of non-adherence to medication regimen is likely greater when patients are instructed to separate levothyroxine doses from food or other medication doses; consistent administration is preferred over the package insert instructions provided (19).

Substances known to reduce levothyroxine absorption should be avoided at the same time of medication doses including calcium and iron supplements, soy products, and antacids. Celiac disease or other disorders of malabsorption or achlorhydria can also reduce medication absorption. Compounded and solution preparations of levothyroxine are not stable and tablet forms are preferred, even in infants and children. Tablets can be chewed or crushed and reconstituted in small amounts of liquid with each administration. Crushed doses should not be dissolved in full serving cups or full bottles of liquids as patients may not consume the complete dose due to incomplete consumption or due to attachment of the dose to the walls of the vessel. Tablets are scored, and ideal dosing may require half doses or combinations of two doses to achieve biochemical euthyroidism.

Generic formulations of levothyroxine are generally equivalent to name brand versions, but in some patients, name brand medication may be preferred. Levothyroxine tablets across manufacturers have consistent colors that match strengths of drug, but shapes and sizes of pills vary between manufacturers. Patients may not always remember their correct dose, but may be able to recall the color of the medicine as a quick guide to knowing the dose they are currently receiving. It is not ideal to switch between generic brand formulation and brand name preparation. Consistency of manufacturer is preferred, otherwise sooner laboratory evaluation may be warranted due to the possible variation of thyroxine quantity between manufacturers.

Liothyronine (LT3) is not indicated in the treatment of acquired hypothyroidism in children and can cause greater likelihood of hyperthyroidism. Likewise, desiccated thyroid hormone products have variable proportions of T3 and T4 and thus can lead to less reliable and consistent thyroid hormone dosing. Despite these preparations having anecdotal claims of superior symptom improvement, no evidence-based research has demonstrated better outcomes over levothyroxine.

NON-THYROIDAL ILLNESS SYNDROME

With the increased ease of thyroid function screening, thyroid lab abnormalities still require explanation in the absence of symptoms. In non-thyroidal illness syndrome, the severity of underlying disease and starvation can result in low T3 and low T4 levels. TSH is low or normal and pituitary and hypothalamic pathology are not likely. Treatment is not usually indicated, and the severity and duration of the underlying illness is reflected in the suppression of the serum thyroxine level (20).

REFERENCES

1. Brown RS. Autoimmune Thyroiditis in Childhood. *J Clin Res Ped Endo* 2013;5(Suppl 1):45–9.
2. Zimmerman MB. Iodine Deficiency. *Endo Rev* 2009;30(4):376–408.
3. Francis GL, Waguespack SG, Bauer AJ, Angelos P, Benvenga S, Cerutti JM, et al. Management Guidelines for Children with Thyroid Nodules and Differentiated Thyroid Cancer. *Thyroid* 2015;25(7):716–59.
4. Reinehr T, de Sousa G, Andler W. Hyperthyrotropinemia in Obese Children Is Reversible after Weight Loss and Is Not Related to Lipids. *J Clin Endo Met* 2006;91(8):3088–91.
5. Matusik P, Gawlik A, Januszek-Trzciakowska A, Malecka-Tendera E. Isolated Subclinical Hyperthyrotropinemia in Obese Children: Does Levothyroxine (LT4) Improve Weight Reduction during Combined Behavioral Therapy? *Int J Endo* 2015;792509.
6. Connelly KJ, Boston BA, Pearce EN, Sesser D, Snyder D, Braverman LE, et al. Congenital Hypothyroidism Caused by Excess Prenatal Maternal Iodine Ingestion. *J Pediatr* 2012;161(4):760–2.
7. Leung AM, Braverman LE. Consequences of Excess Iodine. *Nat Rev Endocrinol* 2014;10(3):136–42.
8. Stinca S, Andersson M, Weibel S, Herter-Aeberli I, Fingerhut R, Gowachirapant S, et al. Dried Blood Spot Thyroglobulin as a Biomarker of Iodine Status in Pregnant Women. *J Clin Endo Met* 2017;102(1):23–32.
9. Ross DS, Burch HB, Cooper DS, Greenlee MC, Laurberg P, Maia AL, et al. American Thyroid Association Guidelines for Diagnosis and Management of Hyperthyroidism and Other Causes of Thyrotoxicosis. *Thyroid* 2016;26(10):1343–421.
10. Shankar RK, Backeljauw PF. Current Best Practice in the Management of Turner Syndrome. *Ther Adv Endo Met* 2018;9(1):33–40.
11. Bull MJ and the Committee on Genetics. Health Supervision for Children with Down Syndrome. *Pediatrics* 2001;107(2).
12. Davis S, Howell S, Wilson R, Tanda T, Ross J, Zeitler P, et al. Advances in the Interdisciplinary Care of Children with Klinefelter Syndrome. *Adv Ped* 2016;63(1):15–46.

13. Haugen BR. Drugs That Suppress TSH or Cause Central Hypothyroidism. *Best Prac Res Clin Endo Meta* 2009;23(6):793–800.
14. Choosingwisely.Org.
15. Rotondi M, de Martinis L, Coperchini F, Pignatti P, Pirali B, Ghilotti S, et al. Serum Negative Autoimmune Thyroiditis Displays a Milder Clinical Picture Compared with Classic Hashimoto's Thyroiditis. *Eur J Endocrinol* 2014;171(1):31–6.
16. Hayashi Y, Tamai H, Fukata S, Hirota Y, Katayama S, Kuma K, et al. A Long Term Clinical, Immunological, and Histological Follow-Up Study of Patients with Goitrous Chronic Lymphocytic Thyroiditis. *J Clin Endo Met* 1985;61(6):1172–8.
17. Jonklaas J, Bianco AC, Bauer AJ, Burman KD, Cappola AR, Celi FS, et al. Guidlines for the Treatment of Hypothyroidism. *Thyroid* 2014;24(12).
18. Svensson J, Ericsson UB, Nilsson P, Olsson C, Jonsson B, Lindberg B, Ivarsson SA. Levothyroxine Treatment Reduces Thyroid Size in Children and Adolescents with Chronic Autoimmune Thyroiditis. *J Clin Endo Met* 2006;91(5):1729–34.
19. Bolk N, Visser TJ, Nijman J, Jongste IJ, Tijssen JG, Berghout A. Effects of Evening vs. Morning Levothyroxine Intake: A Randomized Double-Blind Crossover Trial. *Arch Intern Med* 2010;170(22):1996–2003.
20. DeGroot LJ. The Non-Thyroidal Illness Syndrome. [Updated 2015 Feb 1]. In: Feingold KR, Anawalt B, Boyce A, et al. editors. *Endotext* [Internet]. South Dartmouth (MA): MDText.com.

Hyperthyroidism

SCOTT A. RIVKEES

Several conditions cause hyperthyroidism in childhood (Table 5.1), with Graves' disease (GD) being the most common cause and the primary focus of this chapter. Other causes of hyperthyroidism in children include autonomously functioning thyroid nodules, Hashitoxicosis, neonatal thyrotoxicosis, and infections of the thyroid. Hyperthyroidism also results from thyroid hormone ingestion, McCune–Albright syndrome, struma ovarii, and TSH-producing pituitary adenomas, which are not discussed in this chapter.

EVALUATION OF HYPERTHYROIDISM

Hyperthyroidism can present with overt symptoms, silently, or with isolated thyromegaly (Table 5.2). One of the universal features of hyperthyroidism is tachycardia. Other clinical features can include a prominent stare and proptosis, although eye findings occur less commonly in children than adults.

In hyperthyroidism thyroxine (T4), free T4 (FT4), and/or triiodothyronine (T3) levels are elevated, and thyrotropin (TSH) levels are suppressed. Several

Table 5.1 Causes of hyperthyroidism in childhood

Immune-mediated
Graves' disease
Hashitoxicosis
Infectious thyroiditis
Viral
Bacterial
Adenomas
Toxic adenoma
Multinodular goiter
Abnormal signal transduction
McCune–Albright syndrome
TSH receptor mutations
Increased TSH production
TSH-producing pituitary adenoma
Thyroid hormone resistance
Follicular carcinoma
Medication-induced
Iodine
Amiodarone
Lithium
Exogenous
Excessive levothyroxine intake
Food contamination
Conditions that may be confused for hyperthyroidism
Familial dysalbuminemic hyperthyroxinemia
Thyroid hormone resistance β (RTHβ)

conditions are seen in which thyroid hormone levels are abnormal, yet the individual is euthyroid. Because of their confusing nature, these conditions may result in the patients being erroneously diagnosed or treated for hypothyroidism or hyperthyroidism. When FT4 values are normal, yet total T4 values are high, familial dysalbuminemic hyperthyroxinemia (FDH) needs to be considered. Although FDH can be confused with hyperthyroidism, a distinguishing feature from GD is that TSH levels are not suppressed.

Ultrasensitive TSH assays have been developed and the assessment of TSH by these methods has greatly improved the evaluation of the thyroid status. When both T4 and TSH levels are elevated, TSH-producing pituitary adenomas and thyroid hormone resistance need to be considered. In most truly hyperthyroid states, however, TSH levels are suppressed.

Hyperthyroidism is distinguished from subclinical hyperthyroidism, a condition in which levels of T4, FT4, and T3 are normal, but TSH levels are suppressed.

Table 5.2 Symptoms and signs of
pediatric thyrotoxicosis

Present in more than 50% of children
Tachycardia
Nervousness
Thyromegally
Increased pulse pressure
Hypertension
Tremor
Increased appetite
Weight loss
Thyroid bruit
Present in less than 50% of children
Exophthalmos
Increased perspiration
Hyperactivity
Heart murmur
Palpitations
Heat intolerance
Fatigue
Headache
Diarrhea

The causes of subclinical hyperthyroidism are similar to those of overt hyperthyroidism. Thus, it is important to reevaluate individuals with isolated suppression of TSH levels every 3 to 6 months.

Graves' disease

GD affects 1 in 10,000 children. GD is an autoimmune disorder caused by thyroid gland stimulation by thyroid receptor antibodies (TRAbs; or thyroid-stimulating immunoglobulins [TSI]) and involves genetic factors.

Hyperthyroidism can exert profound adverse effects on children, including excessive physical activity, tremor, tachycardia, flushing, palpitations, weight loss, accelerated linear growth, reduced bone mineralization, premature closure of cranial sutures, and poor school performance. In comparison with adults, eye disease occurs in the minority of pediatric patients with GD, and when it occurs, is usually mild.

Over the past several years additional outcome data have become available to complement older studies looking at spontaneous remission rates of children with GD. Collectively, these studies show that most pediatric patients with GD will not undergo spontaneous remission even after many years of antithyroid drug (ATD) therapy. Thus, most pediatric patients will require either radioactive iodine (^{131}I) or surgery.

ANTITHYROID DRUG THERAPY

ATDs act by inhibiting oxidation and organification of iodide to impair thyroid hormone production and include methimazole (MMI), its precursor carbimazole (CMZ), and propylthiouracil (PTU). MMI is 10 to 20 times more potent than PTU and has a longer half-life. Importantly, these medications do not cure the hyperthyroid state, rather they palliate the condition until spontaneous remission occurs or definitive therapy is rendered. Because it takes 1 or 2 months until biochemical hyperthyroidism resolves on drug therapy, treatment with beta-blockers (propranolol, atenolol, or metoprolol) can be used to control GD symptoms (Table 5.3).

Each of these medications is associated with adverse events that must be considered when prescribed. Before the initiation of drug therapy, a back-up plan that considers the patient's age and treatment risks must be developed at therapy onset in case a toxic reaction occurs. Failure to initially consider alternative treatments can result in a crisis when adverse effects occur.

MMI is now the drug of choice for hyperthyroidism. The MMI doses described in published reports range from 0.1 to 1.0 mg/kg per day (Table 5.3). However, one does not need to use high doses at treatment onset, as MMI side effects are in part dose-related. The response to ATDs influencing circulating thyroid hormone levels is not instantaneous, and several months are needed for thyroid hormone levels to normalize. Thyroid function tests should be obtained monthly after therapy onset. After T4 levels become normal, in most cases the MMI dose can be reduced to minimal doses maintaining euthyroidism. Although MMI is often prescribed in divided doses over the day, once-a-day dosing is sufficient and is associated with better compliance than multiple daily doses.

MMI is available in 5, 10, and 20 mg tablets. When used in children, the following doses that are fractions of tablets can be used: infants, 1.25 mg per day; 1 to 5 years, 2.5 to 5.0 mg/day; 5 to 10 years, 5 to 10 mg/day; and 10 to 18 years, 10 to 20 mg/day. Because the hyperthyroid state can be associated with low white cell counts, and patients will be treated with a medication that can depress neutrophil levels, one should obtain a complete blood count at therapy onset.

Table 5.3 Medical therapy for pediatric GD as related to age

Age	Beta-blocker*	MMI
Newborn	Propranolol, 0.5–1 mg/kg BID	1.25 mg
1 to 5 years	Atenolol or metoprolol, 12.5 mg HS or BID	2.5–5 mg
5 to 10 years	Atenolol or metoprolol, 12.5–25 mg HS or BID	5–10 mg
10 to 15 years	Atenolol or metoprolol, 12.5–25 mg HS or BID	10–15 mg
>15 years	Atenolol or metoprolol, 25 mg HS or BID	10–20 mg

*Atenolol and metoprolol preferred in older individuals. Propranolol preferred in neonates. Doses may be increased by 25% every 2 to 4 days to achieve heart rate in normal range.

MMI therapy is not without risks. Minor side effects may affect up to 20% of children, and major side effects may occur in 1% of children. The most common minor adverse side effects related to MMI are hives, arthralgia, and neutropenia. Children may also develop major side effects, including agranulocytosis, Stevens–Johnson syndrome, and vasculitis. MMI adverse events most commonly occur within 6 months of therapy onset. The agranulocytosis risk is dose-dependent and is rare. If an individual receiving MMI feels ill, becomes febrile, or develops pharyngitis, MMI should be stopped immediately, a practitioner contacted, and a complete blood cell count obtained.

Based on considerable evidence, prolonged ATD therapy will not result in an increased chance of remission for most children, whereas in a minority of children it may. The chance of remission after years of ATDs will be low if the thyroid gland is large (>2 times normal size for age), the child is young (<12 years), not Caucasian, serum TRAb/TSI levels are elevated, or the patient presents with profound hyperthyroidism (FT$_4$ >4 ng/dL).

For children with unfavorable risk factors for spontaneous remission at treatment onset, it is reasonable to treat children for up to 2 years with MMI and see if spontaneous remission occurs. At that point, if there is no remission, it is appropriate to consider definitive therapy if desired by the family. Alternatively, treatment for longer periods can be continued, if side effects to medication do not occur. This approach may be especially useful if the child is considered too young for surgery or radioactive iodine. For the child with favorable risk factors for remission, if spontaneous remission has not occurred after the 2 years of ATDs, continuation of antithyroid medication for prolonged periods is also acceptable, yet one needs to be attentive to adverse effects.

RADIOACTIVE IODINE THERAPY

The goal for ^{131}I therapy for GD is to induce hypothyroidism. Dosages delivering 10,000 to 20,000 cGy to the thyroid are more often used and result in partial or complete destruction of the thyroid. Typically, administered thyroid activities of 150 uCi/g (5.5 MBq/g) generate radiation doses of 12,000 cGy to the thyroid. Dosing is based on the Quimby–Marinelli equation: dose (β + γ radiation; in Gy) = 90 × (oral iodine-131 dose [μCi] × oral 24-hour uptake [%]/g × 100%). For example, if the desired dosage is 300 uCi/g, and the thyroid is 30 grams with an uptake of 75% (0.75), the desired administered dosage will be 12 mCi. (Dosage in mCi = 300 uCi/g × 30 g/ 0.75 uptake = 12,000 uCi or 12 mCi.)

Some centers give a fixed administered dosage of 10 or 15 mCi ^{131}I to all children, rather than individually calculated activities. There are no studies comparing outcomes of fixed vs. calculated activities in children. In adults, the two different approaches lead to similar outcomes; however, in children, there is a potential advantage of calculated vs. fixed dosing.

When children are to be treated with ^{131}I, ATDs should be stopped 3 to 5 days prior to treatment. Patients are placed on beta-blockers until T4 and/or FT4 levels normalize post-therapy. Whereas some clinicians restart ATDs after treatment with ^{131}I, this is rarely required in children. Thyroid hormone levels begin to decrease about 7 days after radioiodine therapy in children. Continued ATD use can make it difficult to assess if post-treatment hypothyroidism is the result of ^{131}I or the ATD.

There are rare reports of children with severe hyperthyroidism developing thyroid storm after [131]I. In general, these children were severely hyperthyroid when ^{131}I was administered. Thus, if T4 levels are >20 µg/dl or FT4 levels are >5 ng/dl, children should be treated with MMI until T4 and/or free T4 levels normalize before proceeding with ^{131}I therapy. Importantly, most children with GD have been hyperthyroid for months prior to diagnosis and there is no need to rush to ^{131}I therapy.

It usually takes 6 to 12 weeks after ^{131}I treatment for the patient to become biochemically euthyroid or hypothyroid. Until then, symptoms of hyperthyroidism can be controlled using beta-blockers. The use of SSKI (saturated solution of potassium iodide) or Lugol's solution 1 week after ^{131}I will also quickly attenuate biochemical hyperthyroidism without adversely affecting the outcome of radioiodine therapy.

The development of progression of ophthalmopathy following ^{131}I in adults has been reported. However, children rarely develop severe ophthalmopathy and proptosis is mild. Studies show that eye disease worsens in only a small percentage of children with GD, irrespective of therapy type.

In adults, it has been shown that progression of ophthalmopathy can be prevented by treatment with prednisone for 3 months following ^{131}I therapy. Adjunctive prednisone therapy is not routinely recommended for most children, as most do not have significant eye disease. The prolonged administration of prednisone is also associated with growth failure, weight gain, and immune suppression. Nevertheless, prednisone (0.5 mg/kg × 4–6 weeks) may be useful for the child who has moderate or severe eye disease and will be treated with [131]I.

There is no evidence showing adverse effects to offspring of children treated with [131]I. Birth defects are not higher in offspring born to individuals treated with ^{131}I for hyperthyroidism during childhood or adolescence.

The risk of thyroid neoplasms in children is greatest with exposure to low-level external radiation (0.1–25 Gy; ~0.09–30 uCi/g) and not with the higher activities used to treat GD. At present, we are not aware of any cases of thyroid cancer that developed in pediatric patients treated with >150 uCi of ^{131}I per gram of thyroid tissue for childhood GD that can be attributed to ^{131}I therapy.

Important in considering radioactive iodine use in children are the potential influences of ^{131}I therapy on other cancers, as ^{131}I therapy results in low-level, whole-body radiation exposure. Several studies in adults have examined potential risks of ^{131}I therapy for GD on cancers. These studies have not revealed increased mortality or increased rates of cancer following ^{131}I for GD. Based on theoretical calculations of potential cancer risk after ^{131}I, we feel that it is prudent to avoid radioactive iodine therapy in children under 5 years of age and to avoid >10 mCi in patients younger than 10 years old.

THYROIDECTOMY

Surgery is an effective form of therapy for GD if it can be performed by an expert surgeon and in some situations is preferable to radioactive iodine. When surgery is performed, near-total or total thyroidectomy is indicated, as subtotal thyroidectomy is associated with a higher relapse rate. Hypothyroidism is nearly universal in children and adults who undergo total thyroidectomy. In comparison, after subtotal thyroidectomy, hyperthyroidism recurs in 10–15% of patients.

Surgery is preferred in children younger than 5 years when definitive therapy is needed and can be performed by a skilled, high-volume thyroid surgeon. In individuals who have large thyroid glands (>80 g), the response to ^{131}I is poor, and surgery is recommended for these patients.

In preparation for surgery, the patient should be rendered euthyroid. Typically, this is done by continuing MMI until T4 levels normalize. A week before surgery, iodine drops are started (1–3 drops, t.i.d.), which inhibits thyroid hormone production and causes the gland to become firm and less vascular.

Postoperatively, younger pediatric patients are at a higher risk for transient hypoparathyroidism than adolescents or adults. To mitigate postoperative hypocalcemia, children may be treated with 50,000 U of vitamin D 1 week before surgery or with calcitriol. Complication rates are related to the expertise of surgeon. Considering these data, if local pediatric thyroid surgery expertise is unavailable, referral of a child with GD to a high-volume, thyroid surgery center with pediatric experience should be considered. Very low complication rates for children undergoing thyroidectomy for GD have been reported with this type of multidisciplinary model.

NEONATAL THYROTOXICOSIS

Thyrotoxicosis in the neonate is a severe and life-threatening condition that can be associated with lasting neurologic problems. Neonatal thyrotoxicosis most commonly occurs in the setting of active or past maternal GD. The risk of fetal hyperthyroidism and neonatal GD is proportional to the magnitude of elevation of TRAb levels. Fetal hyperthyroidism is generally associated with levels of TRAbs more than two to four times greater than the upper limit of normal for assay. Because the fetus is at risk for hyperthyroidism when there is active or past maternal GD, fetal growth and heart rate should be regularly assessed from mid-pregnancy onward. Excessive fetal heart rate (>160 beats per minute after 20 weeks) and the presence of a fetal goiter suggest hyperthyroidism in the fetus. In addition, accelerated maturation of the femoral ossification center is seen with fetal hyperthyroidism.

If a mother with a history of GD is not taking ATDs during pregnancy, the fetus may develop intrauterine hyperthyroidism. If fetal hyperthyroidism is recognized prenatally by the presence of fetal tachycardia (heart rate higher than 160 beats per minute after 22 weeks), treatment of the mother with antithyroid drugs will reduce intrauterine thyrotoxicosis.

Treatment of thyrotoxic infants consists of administration of MMI (1.25 mg per day) and beta-blockers (propranolol 1 mg per kg per day). Lugol's solution or SSKI may be given (1 to 2 drops every 8 hours) for 7 to 10 days to more rapidly control biochemical hyperthyroidism. After approximately 2 weeks of antithyroid drug therapy, thyroid hormone levels will decline. When thyroid hormone levels fall below normal, supplementary levothyroxine (37.5 μg per day for full-term infants) is added to prevent hypothyroidism. As TRAbs are cleared from the infant's circulation, spontaneous recovery begins within 3 months and is usually complete by 6 months. Thus, the infant can be weaned from treatment after 3 months. Monitoring of the infant's TRAb levels is also a useful predictor of when antithyroid medication can be tapered.

HASHITOXICOSIS

Uncommonly, thyrotoxicosis is an initial thyrotoxic phase in patients with Hashimoto's thyroiditis in which immunologic destruction of thyroid tissue results in the release of preformed thyroid hormone, which leads to elevated T4 levels. In contrast to GD, hyperthyroidism is transient, eye findings are absent, radionuclide uptake is low, and elevated levels of thyroid-stimulating immunoglobulins are not present. This condition can be distinguished from GD by low uptake within the thyroid gland of radionuclides and its transient nature, lasting a few months. Some reserve the term Hashitoxicosis for patients with autoimmune thyroid disease who present with phases of GD and hypothyroidism associated with stimulating and blocking thyroid autoantibodies.

HYPERFUNCTIONING THYROID NODULES

Warm or hot nodules lead to excessive production of thyroid hormone and can be associated with clinical and biochemical hyperthyroidism. Interestingly, activating somatic mutations of the TSH receptor and G_s have been discovered in hyperfunctioning nodules. Although hyperfunctioning nodules may be ablated with radioiodine, surgical excision of hyperfunctioning nodules is recommended in children and adolescents, because radiation-exposed normal thyroid tissue will remain after the hyperfunctioning nodule is ablated. Alternatively, one can consider thermal ablation (radiofrequency, laser). Although the risk of malignancy in hyperfunctioning nodules is low, thyroid cancers have been described in warm nodules.

Infectious bacterial thyroiditis

Occasionally a child presents with hyperthyroidism, tenderness over the thyroid gland, and fever due to bacterial infection of the thyroid, a condition called acute thyroiditis. Acute thyroiditis can be associated with the presence of a fistula connecting the piriform sinus on the left side of the pharynx to the thyroid. Fevers can be high, and erythrocyte sedimentation rates and white counts elevated. Ultrasonography may reveal a local abscess. In contrast to GD, uptake of technetium 99-pertechnetate or radioiodine is reduced when thyroid scanning is performed.

The offending bacteria include *Hemophilus influenza* and group A streptococci. Thus, treatment with an antibiotic resistant to disruption by beta-lactamase is recommended. In severe cases, hospitalization and intravenous antibiotic administration is indicated, because lymphatic drainage into the mediastinal region may occur. Surgical drainage is needed if a localized abscess develops and the response to antibiotics is poor.

Because the infectious process results in destruction of thyroid tissue, release of preformed thyroid hormone and hyperthyroidism may occur during infection. The hyperthyroid state is usually transient, and treatment with antithyroid drugs is not indicated. If the patient becomes symptomatic, beta-blockers may be used.

After the child has recovered, pharyngography is indicated to test for a patent piriform sinus tract. Occasionally, the tract may close as the result of the infection. If the tract persists, however, and acute thyroiditis recurs, resection is needed.

Summary

Thyrotoxicosis can have profound effects on the fetus, neonate, child, and adolescent. The causes of hyperthyroidism can be distinguished by clinical and diagnostic features. Fortunately, effective treatments are available for the vast majority of conditions that result in hyperthyroidism in the pediatric population.

SELECTED REFERENCES

Ross DS, Burch HB, Cooper DS, Greenlee MC, Laurberg P, Maia AL, et al. 2016 American Thyroid Association Guidelines for Diagnosis and Management of Hyperthyroidism and Other Causes of Thyrotoxicosis. *Thyroid* 2016;26(10):1343–421.

Rivkees SA. Controversies in the Management of Graves' Disease in Children. *J Endocrinol Invest* 2016;39(11):1247–57.

Rivkees SA, Cornelius EA. Influence of Iodine-131 Dose on the Outcome of Hyperthyroidism in Children. *Pediatrics* 2003;111(4 Pt 1):745–9.

Bauer AJ. Thyroid Nodules in Children and Adolescents. *Curr Opin Endocrinol Diabetes Obes* 2019;26(5):266–74.

Baumgarten HD, Bauer AJ, Isaza A, Mostoufi-Moab S, Kazahaya K, Adzick NS. Surgical Management of Pediatric Thyroid Disease: Complication Rates After Thyroidectomy at the Children's Hospital of Philadelphia High-Volume Pediatric Thyroid Center. *J Pediatr Surg* 2019;54(10):1969–75.

Samuels SL, Namoc SM, Bauer AJ. Neonatal Thyrotoxicosis. *Clin Perinatol* 2018;45(1):31–40.

6

Thyroid nodules

CATHERINE McMANUS, JENNIFER H. KUO, AND
JAMES A. LEE

INTRODUCTION

In 2009, the American Thyroid Association (ATA) published a single set of guidelines on the management of thyroid nodules for both children and adults (1). However, as more data regarding the implications and malignant potential of thyroid nodules among children became available, the difference between thyroid nodules in a child vs. an adult became more distinct. Thus, a separate set of guidelines for the management of thyroid nodules among children was published by the ATA in 2015, noting important differences in the workup and management of thyroid nodules in the pediatric population (2).

PREVALENCE

Thyroid nodules are less common in children compared to adults. According to studies focusing on imaging or postmortem examinations, thyroid nodules occur with a frequency of only 1–1.5% among children and 13% among adolescences (3). In contrast, the prevalence of thyroid nodules in adults can be as high as 65% depending on age (4). While less common in children, pediatric thyroid nodules have a greater risk of malignancy at approximately 22–26% compared to the 5% of nodules that carry malignancy among adults (5, 6).

RISK FACTORS

Similar to the adult population, risk factors for the development of thyroid nodules in the pediatric population include radiation exposure, iodine deficiency, and a history of thyroid disease. Among children, radiation exposure poses the greatest risk for development of thyroid nodules and thyroid cancer (7, 8). Specifically, childhood cancer survivors who were treated with radiation develop thyroid nodules at a rate of 2% per year, which reaches a peak incidence up to 25 years after exposure (9, 10). Studies have demonstrated that the risk is greatest for those who received higher doses of radiation (up to 20–29 Gy) before reaching 15 years of age (8, 11).

Another risk factor for the development of thyroid nodules in children is autoimmune thyroiditis. Up to 30% of children with autoimmune thyroiditis are found to have thyroid nodules, with a 23% rate of malignancy according to one study by Corrias et al. in 2008 (12). Similar to the adult population, the number of incidentally discovered thyroid nodules that would have reached clinical significance, even among high-risk patients, is unknown. However, there is a lower threshold to do further workup of a thyroid nodule in a child given the higher rate of malignancy.

EVALUATION

A palpable thyroid nodule, a diffusely enlarged thyroid gland, and/or cervical lymphadenopathy that is noted on physical exam in a child warrants evaluation with thyroid function testing and a formal neck ultrasound. The ultrasound should include evaluation of the thyroid gland as well as for the presence or absence of cervical lymphadenopathy (2).

Hyperfunctioning thyroid nodules

If laboratory workup reveals a suppressed TSH, a nuclear medicine radioisotope scan should be performed to assess for a hyperfunctioning thyroid nodule. Children with toxic adenomas, characterized by a focal increase in uptake on the radioisotope scan, may have mild signs and symptoms of hyperthyroidism or may be euthyroid. Studies have suggested that up to 30% of children with a hyperfunctioning nodule have differentiated thyroid cancer (2, 13). Thus, if workup reveals a hyperfunctioning thyroid nodule, the recommended approach is to proceed directly to surgical resection. While alternative therapies for toxic adenomas exist in the adult population, including radioactive iodine ablation or ethanol injection, these techniques are not well studied in children. Furthermore, the higher risk of malignancy and the theoretical concern of low-activity radioiodine causing mutagenesis on normal thyroid tissue preclude less invasive therapies for a toxic adenoma in the pediatric population at this time (2).

Nonfunctional thyroid nodules

If the TSH is not suppressed, workup should proceed by determining if a fine needle aspiration biopsy (FNAB) is warranted. Similar to the revised 2015 ATA guidelines for adults, the 2015 ATA recommendations for the pediatric population note that the size of the nodule is less predictive of malignancy compared to ultrasound characteristics. This is especially true in children, since the thyroid volume changes with age. Thus, the decision to perform an FNAB of a nodule should be based on imaging characteristics, which are discussed in a separate chapter (2, 14, 15). If a FNAB is warranted based on imaging characteristics, the biopsy should be performed under ultrasound guidance (2).

Diffusely enlarged thyroid gland

One important difference in the pediatric population is the evaluation of a diffusely enlarged thyroid gland. In children, papillary thyroid carcinoma can potentially present as a diffuse infiltrating disease that involves the entire lobe or gland. The majority of diffusely infiltrating PTC will have microcalcifications on ultrasound; thus, all children with a diffusely enlarged thyroid gland should undergo an ultrasound and subsequent biopsy if microcalcifications are noted (2).

Screening ultrasound

Although there is an increase in the prevalence of thyroid nodules among high-risk children, such as those with a history of radiation exposure or autoimmune thyroiditis, it is not well demonstrated that a screening ultrasound and subsequent FNAB lead to improvement in quality or duration of life (16). Consequently, there are no formal recommendations for screening ultrasound among high-risk children at this time (2).

THE BETHESDA SYSTEM

The analysis of thyroid nodules for children and adults utilizes the Bethesda System for Reporting Thyroid Cytopathology (17). Nodules can be placed into one of six categories including non-diagnostic or unsatisfactory (Bethesda I), benign

(Bethesda II), atypia of undetermined significance (AUS), or follicular lesion of undetermined significance (FLUS) (Bethesda III), suspicious for follicular or Hürthle cell neoplasm (Bethesda IV), suspicious for malignancy (Bethesda V), or malignant (Bethesda VI). However, there are important differences between children and adults in the prevalence of malignancy as well as the recommended management for each category (Table 6.1).

Bethesda I

When the FNA result is non-diagnostic or unsatisfactory (Bethesda I), the risk of malignancy among adults is 1–4%. However, the exact risk of malignancy among children with a non-diagnostic FNA is not well studied. The recommendation for both children and adults is to have a repeat FNA biopsy; however, one should wait at least 3 months to repeat the biopsy in children to avoid the possibility for atypical cells that may occur in the remodeling process (18). If the repeat biopsy is non-diagnostic, options include repeating an ultrasound in 6 months if the nodule is stable in size and ultrasound characteristics, or lobectomy (2).

Bethesda II

The recommendation for a benign Bethesda II nodule is to observe, given that the rate of false negative biopsies among children and adults is only 3–5% (19). Repeat ultrasound is recommended every 1–2 years, with a repeat biopsy if the nodule increases in size or develops suspicious characteristics. Once a nodule reaches 4 cm, surgery should be considered if there are solid features present (2).

Table 6.1 The Bethesda System for reporting thyroid cytopathology in children

	Diagnostic category	Risk of malignancy (%)	Management
I	Nondiagnostic or unsatisfactory	1–4	Repeat biopsy
II	Benign	0–3	Observation
III	Atypia of undetermined significance (AUS) or follicular lesion of undetermined significance (FLUS)	18–28	Lobectomy
IV	Follicular neoplasm or suspicious for a follicular neoplasm	58	Lobectomy
V	Suspicious for malignancy	75–100	Total thyroidectomy
VI	Malignant	99–100	Total thyroidectomy

Bethesda III/IV

A Bethesda III result, which indicates atypia or a follicular lesion of undetermined significance (AUS/FLUS), carries a risk of malignancy of 18–28% in children. In contrast, Bethesda III carries a risk of malignancy of 6–18% in adults if noninvasive follicular thyroid neoplasm with papillary-like nuclear factors (NIFTP) is excluded from the malignancy category (17, 20). For children with a Bethesda IV result (suspicious for follicular neoplasm) the risk of malignancy is as high as 58%, compared to 10–40% among adults if NIFTP is excluded from malignancy (17, 21, 22). Given the higher risk of malignancy in children, a lobectomy with isthmusectomy is recommended for Bethesda III and Bethesda IV nodules (21).

Bethesda V/VI

The Bethesda V and Bethesda VI categories are used when cytologic features are suspicious for malignancy or conclusive for malignancy, respectively. The rates of malignancy for pediatric patients in these two categories are reported to be 100%; however, the sample sizes in these studies are small (20, 23). Consequently, it is reasonable to apply the risk of malignancy in adults for categories V and VI, up to 60% and up to 96%, respectively (excluding NIFTP from malignancies) (17). Thyroid nodules with a Bethesda V or VI category warrant total thyroidectomy in children (2, 24).

MOLECULAR PROFILING

Perhaps the greatest difference between children and adults regarding thyroid nodules is the management of an indeterminate FNA result. For adults, the recommended management of indeterminate nodules includes a repeat FNA biopsy, a diagnostic lobectomy, or further evaluation of the nodule with molecular profiling. Over the last 20 years, there has been a significant expansion in the understanding of molecular genomics that has led to the development of diagnostic testing that can identify which indeterminate nodules are at a higher risk of cancer and should be removed (24).

In a study by Monaco et al., 17% of nodules in the pediatric population had an FNA that was positive for a mutation and ultimately was diagnosed as malignant. Thus, a positive mutation has a high correlation with malignancy; however, the Bethesda classification for those nodules included Bethesda III–VI, all of which would have led to surgical resection in the pediatric population given the higher rates of malignancy for these categories (21, 24).

Furthermore, molecular profiling can help identify which nodules can be safely observed among adults. While these tests may be useful in the pediatric population to possibly avoid surgery for a benign nodule, further studies are necessary to validate gene expression classifiers among children in order to reliably exclude malignancy (25).

CONCLUSION

The ATA first published a set of guidelines for the management of pediatric thyroid nodules in 2015, noting important differences between children and adults. While thyroid nodules are less common in children compared to adults, the risk of malignancy is higher. Therefore, a more aggressive approach that includes diagnostic lobectomy for indeterminate nodules and total thyroidectomy for nodules that are suspicious for or confirmed malignancy is recommended. Finally, validation studies in the pediatric population are needed prior to the implementation of nonsurgical techniques for hyperfunctioning nodules and molecular profiling for indeterminate nodules.

REFERENCES

1. Cooper DS, Doherty GM, Haugen BR, Kloos RT, Lee SL, Mandel SJ, et al. Revised American Thyroid Association Management Guidelines for Patients with Thyroid Nodules and Differentiated Thyroid Cancer. *Thyroid* 2009;19(11):1167–214.
2. Francis GL, Waguespack SG, Bauer AJ, Angelos P, Benvenga S, Cerutti JM, et al. Management Guidelines for Children with Thyroid Nodules and Differentiated Thyroid Cancer. *Thyroid* 2015;25(7):716–59.
3. Niedziela M, Korman E, Breborowicz D, Trejster E, Harasymczuk J, Warzywoda M, et al. A Prospective Study of Thyroid Nodular Disease in Children and Adolescents in Western Poland from 1996 to 2000 and the Incidence of Thyroid Carcinoma Relative to Iodine Deficiency and the Chernobyl Disaster. *Pediatr Blood Cancer* 2004;42(1):84–92.
4. Haugen BR, Alexander EK, Bible KC, Doherty GM, Mandel SJ, Nikiforov YE, et al. 2015 American Thyroid Association Management Guidelines for Adult Patients with Thyroid Nodules and Differentiated Thyroid Cancer: The American Thyroid Association Guidelines Task Force on Thyroid Nodules and Differentiated Thyroid Cancer. *Thyroid* 2016;26(1):1–133.
5. Gupta A, Ly S, Castroneves LA, Frates MC, Benson CB, Feldman HA, et al. A Standardized Assessment of Thyroid Nodules in Children Confirms Higher Cancer Prevalence than in Adults. *J Clin Endocrinol Metab* 2013;98(8):3238–45.
6. Niedziela M. Pathogenesis, Diagnosis and Management of Thyroid Nodules in Children. *Endocr Relat Cancer* 2006;13(2):427–53.
7. Sklar C, Whitton J, Mertens A, Stovall M, Green D, Marina N, et al. Abnormalities of the Thyroid in Survivors of Hodgkin's Disease: Data from the Childhood Cancer Survivor Study. *J Clin Endocrinol Metab* 2000;85(9):3227–32.
8. Meadows AT, Friedman DL, Neglia JP, Mertens AC, Donaldson SS, Stovall M, et al. Second Neoplasms in Survivors of Childhood Cancer: Findings from the Childhood Cancer Survivor Study Cohort. *J Clin Oncol* 2009;27(14):2356–62.

9. Schneider AB, Bekerman C, Leland J, Rosengarten J, Hyun H, Collins B, et al. Thyroid Nodules in the Follow-Up of Irradiated Individuals: Comparison of Thyroid Ultrasound with Scanning and Palpation. *J Clin Endocrinol Metab* 1997;82(12):4020–7.

10. Ito M, Yamashita S, Ashizawa K, Namba H, Hoshi M, Shibata Y et al. Childhood Thyroid Diseases Around Chernobyl Evaluated by Ultrasound Examination and Fine Needle Aspiration Cytology. *Thyroid* 1995;5(5):365–8.

11. Ronckers CM, Sigurdson AJ, Stovall M, Smith SA, Mertens AC, Liu Y, et al. Thyroid Cancer in Childhood Cancer Survivors: A Detailed Evaluation of Radiation Dose Response and its Modifiers. *Radiat Res* 2006;166(4):618–28.

12. Corrias A, Cassio A, Weber G, Mussa A, Wasniewska M, Rapa A, et al. Thyroid Nodules and Cancer in Children and Adolescents Affected by Autoimmune Thyroiditis. *Arch Pediatr Adolesc Med* 2008;162(6):526–31.

13. Niedziela M, Breborowicz D, Trejster E, Korman E. Hot Nodules in Children and Adolescents in Western Poland from 1996 to 2000: Clinical Analysis of 31 Patients. *J Pediatr Endocrinol Metab* 2002;15(6):823–30.

14. Lyshchik A, Drozd V, Demidchik Y, Reiners C. Diagnosis of Thyroid Cancer in Children: Value of Gray-Scale and Power Doppler US. *Radiology*. 2005;235(2):604–13.

15. Drozd VM, Lushchik ML, Polyanskaya ON, Fridman MV, Demidchik YE, Lyshchik AP, et al. The Usual Ultrasonographic Features of Thyroid Cancer are Less Frequent in Small Tumors that Develop After a Long Latent Period after the Chernobyl Radiation Release Accident. *Thyroid* 2009;19(7):725–34.

16. Hayashida N, Imaizumi M, Shimura H, Furuya F, Okubo N, Asari Y, et al. Thyroid Ultrasound Findings in a Follow-Up Survey of Children from Three Japanese Prefectures: Aomori, Yamanashi, and Nagasaki. *Sci Rep*. 2015;5:1–5.

17. Cibas ES, Ali SZ. The 2017 Bethesda System for Reporting Thyroid Cytopathology. *Thyroid* 2017;27(11):1341–6.

18. Baloch ZW, LiVolsi VA. Post Fine-Needle Aspiration Histologic Alterations of Thyroid Revisited. *Am J Clin Pathol* 1999;112(3):311–6.

19. Stevens C, Lee JKP, Sadatsafavi M, Blair GK. Pediatric Thyroid Fine-Needle Aspiration Cytology: A Meta-analysis. *J Pediatr Surg* [Internet]. 2009;44(11):2184–91. doi:10.1016/j.jpedsurg.2009.07.022.

20. Norlén O, Charlton A, Sarkis LM, Henwood T, Shun A, Gill AJ, Delbridge L. Risk of Malignancy for Each Bethesda Class in Pediatric Thyroid Nodules. *J Pediatr Surg* 2015;50(7):1147–9. doi:10.1016/j.jpedsurg.2014.10.046.

21. Monaco SE, Pantanowitz L, Khalbuss WE, Benkovich VA, Ozolek J, Nikiforova MN, et al. Cytomorphological and Molecular Genetic Findings in Pediatric Thyroid Fine-Needle Aspiration. *Cancer Cytopathol* 2012;120(5):342–50.

22. Smith M, Pantanowitz L, Khalbuss WE, Benkovich VA, Monaco SE. Indeterminate Pediatric Thyroid Fine Needle Aspirations: A Study of 68 Cases. *Acta Cytol* 2013;57(4):341–8.
23. Pantola C, Kala S, Khan L, Pantola S, Singh M, Verma S. Cytological Diagnosis of Pediatric Thyroid Nodule in Perspective of the Bethesda System for Reporting Thyroid Cytopathology. *J Cytol* 2016;33(4):220–3.
24. Kuo JH, McManus C, Graves CE, Madani A, Khokhar MT, Huang B, Lee JA. Updates in the Management of Thyroid Nodules. *Curr Probl Surg* [Internet]. 2019;56(3):103–27. doi:10.1067/j.cpsurg.2018.12.003.
25. Alexander EK, Kennedy GC, Baloch ZW, Cibas ES, Chudova D, Diggans J, et al. Preoperative Diagnosis of Benign Thyroid Nodules with Indeterminate Cytology. *N Engl J Med* 2012;367(8):705–15.

7

Thyroid cancer

PALLAVI IYER

PEDIATRIC THYROID CANCER

Pediatric thyroid cancer accounts for 1.5% of all cancers in children younger than 15 years (2 cases per million), but in adolescents 15–19 years of age, it accounts for 8% of all cancer (occurring at a rate of 17 cases per million). The most common histology is papillary (81.8%), follicular (10.1%), and then medullary (8.1%) (undifferentiated thyroid cancers are rare in childhood) based on the National Cancer Institute's Surveillance Epidemiology and End Results (SEER) database between 2007 and 2012(1). In the older age group, there is a female to male preponderance (4.4:1) and papillary and follicular cancers become more likely compared with medullary thyroid carcinoma. Risk factors for developing thyroid cancer in childhood include previous exposure to radiation to the thyroid gland, genetic predisposition conditions, and autoimmune thyroiditis (2) (Figure 7.1).

PAPILLARY THYROID CANCER (PTC)

In children, PTC often presents as multifocal, bilateral, and with regional nodal metastases compared to adults. Despite this extensive nature at presentation, children with PTC have less than 2% long-term cause-specific mortality due to the PTC. The histologic subtypes include classical, solid, follicular, and diffuse sclerosing, tall cell variants with associated level of aggressiveness (2).

Management strategies for PTC

- Total thyroidectomy—with/without central neck dissection (to be covered in the surgical management section)
- Risk stratification postoperative staging about 6 weeks after surgery
- TSH suppression with levothyroxine based on risk level
- Radioactive iodine therapy (RAI) (I-131) based on risk level
- Long-term surveillance with thyroglobulin (Tg) levels, thyroid ultrasound, +/– thyroid uptake and scan; management of surgical complications such as hypoparathyroidism, vocal cord dysfunction
- Consideration for other forms of therapy for metastatic disease including repeated I-131, external beam radiation, surgical resection, and with adjuvant therapies such as tyrosine kinase inhibitors

RISK STRATIFICATION

Based on the American Joint Committee on Cancer (AJCC) tumor, lymph nodes, metastases (TNM) classification system's nodal and distant metastases staging, risk levels can be assigned. The **low-risk group** is defined as tumor grossly confined to the thyroid gland. The **intermediate-risk** group (those with nodal metastasis to central or lateral retropharyngeal lymph nodes) have low risk for distant metastasis, but may have increased risk for persistent cervical disease. Those with extensive lateral nodal disease or locally invasive disease (past the thyroid capsule) are considered the **highest-risk** for incomplete resection, persistent disease of the neck, and distant metastases (2).

THYROID-STIMULATING HORMONE (TSH) SUPPRESSION

The goal of levothyroxine therapy postoperatively is to replace thyroid hormone after thyroidectomy and to suppress thyroid cell growth by suppressing TSH. Thyroglobulin (Tg) is a thyroid-specific, TSH-responsive protein that is made and secreted by normal and differentiated thyroid carcinoma tissue and serves as a sensitive marker for thyroid tissue. Based on the risk level, the goal of therapy for TSH values can be liberalized: for low-risk patients, enough thyroid hormone given (usually 1.7–2 mcg/kg/day) to suppress TSH to 0.5–1.0 mIU/L; for intermediate-risk patients, TSH of 0.1–0.5 mIU/L; and in high-risk patients, TSH of <0.1 mIU/L. A suppressed Tg is also obtained at the 6 weeks mark to assess if further gross thyroid tissue should be assessed for prior to I-131 therapy (2).

NECK ULTRASOUND

If the Tg is elevated after 6–12 weeks, consideration should be given to reassessing the presence of residual tumor (remnant thyroid or loco-regional disease tissue) via a neck ultrasound. A re-operation to remove any such tissue should be considered prior to RAI.

RAI (I-131) THERAPY

Previously, radioactive iodine therapy was recommended for all patients with papillary thyroid carcinoma. Given the low risk of mortality, but perhaps an increased risk of other malignancies with radioactive iodine therapy, we now reserve I-131 therapy for patients in intermediate- to high-risk categories.

To prepare for I-131 therapy, the patient should have levothyroxine discontinued for 2–3 weeks to stimulate the TSH above 30 mIU/L. Alternatively, preparation with recombinant thyrotropin (rhTSH) injection 0.1 mg intramuscularly every 24 hours × 2 may be used in patients who are unable to tolerate a hypothyroid state. A low-iodine diet preceding the I-131 therapy seems to potentiate the uptake of I-131 in the thyroid tissue. It is important that a negative pregnancy test is documented in all post-pubertal girls prior to therapy as I-131 therapy is teratogenic. A stimulated Tg (Tg obtained when TSH is above 30 mIU/L) acts as a tumor marker.

An I-123 or low-dose I-131 scan is performed to assess the extent of cervical disease/lung/bone metastases. If there is gross disease in the nodes identified, a thyroid ultrasound and subsequent surgical consultation should be considered prior to I-131 therapy.

Generally, in pediatric patients, empiric dosing of I-131 based on adjusted body weight (patient's weight/70 kg) or body surface area based on typical adult dosing or (1.0–1.5 mCi/kg) is administered. Dosimetry may be reserved for those with repeated I-131 therapy, concerns for bone marrow suppression, or those with extensive pulmonary metastases (2). Other considerations in preparation for RAI in children is to assess and prepare patients/families for the ability to swallow the radioactive capsule easily, the ability to remain isolated with minimal interaction with others for 24–48 hours, the ability to hydrate adequately, and to have appropriate conditions at home (away from pregnant women and small infants) once discharged. A post I-131 whole-body scan is recommended to identify any residual uptake distantly.

LONG-TERM SURVEILLANCE

Surveillance includes ultrasonography of the neck, Tg measurements (both suppressed and TSH-stimulated), and diagnostic I-123 scans for those with no evidence of disease. Tg should be measured on levothyroxine therapy every 3–6 months initially to look for trends. In low-risk patients, Tg can be measured annually after 2 years without any rise in Tg. In patients in the intermediate-risk and high-risk categories, measurements can be changed to annually after 3 years and a TSH-stimulated Tg with/without a diagnostic I-123 scan could be considered 1–2 years after surgery. A detectable suppressed Tg or stimulated-Tg >2 ng/mL is associated with increased risk of residual disease (2).

A thyroid ultrasound 6 months postoperatively and then 6–12 months for the next 5 years based on the level of risk and concern is also recommended. Children with PTC are most likely to have residual or recurrent disease occur in the associated cervical lymph nodes. If such tissue is identified, an FNA should be performed followed by surgery, if amenable, to resect any disease.

Metastatic disease

Most children with metastatic disease have pulmonary metastases with micronodular disease that tends to be iodine avid. Thus repeated treatments with I-131 and long-term follow-up lead either to resolution of disease or stable disease (i.e., stable Tg levels). If stable disease is present, repeated I-131 treatment for iodide avid disease should be taken with caution given a higher propensity in children to develop iodide-induced pulmonary fibrosis. If I-131 therapy is warranted, dosimetry should be employed to limit exposure to normal lung parenchyma.

In children who have progressive or symptomatic disease not amenable to further surgery or I-131 therapy, considerations for using tyrosine kinase inhibitors could be made in conjunction with oncologists.

FOLLICULAR THYROID CANCER (FTC)

Follicular carcinomas occur less frequently in children and adolescents, occurring with a more equal ratio between males and females compared with papillary thyroid carcinoma. Risk factors worldwide include iodine deficiency and genetic lesions such as *PTEN* hamartoma tumor syndrome (such as Cowden syndrome). The FNA of these lesions show Bethesda Class 3 or 4 (atypia of undetermined significance/follicular lesion of undetermined significance or follicular neoplasm/suspicious for follicular neoplasm). Based on these findings, in children, a lobectomy or total thyroidectomy should be performed by a high-volume surgeon. The diagnosis can only be made on surgical pathology with findings of vascular invasion or capsular invasion.

The care for patients with FTC depends on the findings at the initial diagnosis. Surgical pathology can help differentiate the FTC into two categories: (1) *minimally invasive* with low risk for recurrence or metastases, or (2) *widely invasive FTC* marked with increased morbidity and mortality. Minimally invasive FTC usually is (1) unifocal; (2) unlikely to spread loco-regionally to the nodes; (3) associated with excellent prognosis (2). This can be treated with only lobectomy and followed accordingly (3). Whereas widely invasive FTC is usually (1) 4 cm or larger on initial presentation; (2) invasion of 3 blood vessels or more; (3) more likely to spread hematogenously. Patients with minimally invasive disease could undergo a lobectomy + isthmusectomy without having a second completion surgery. However, in widely invasive FTC, complete thyroidectomy with postoperative staging and consideration for I-131 therapy if postoperative staging shows a stimulated thyroglobulin >10 ng/dL should be considered (3). Surveillance with neck ultrasonography is only needed for those who underwent lobectomy alone, but not with total thyroidectomy as FTC does not tend to spread to regional lymph nodes.

Medullary thyroid carcinoma (MTC)

In children, MTC is generally part of an inherited syndrome—multiple endocrine neoplasia type 2 (MEN 2). Unlike papillary or follicular carcinoma, MTC arises from para-follicular c-cells of the thyroid gland. This tissue secretes calcitonin which serves as a marker for c-cell hyperplasia and carcinoma. MTC also secretes carcinogenic embryonic antigen (CEA) (and less frequently ACTH). MEN results from activating mutations in germline *RET* (*RE*- arranged during transfection) proto-oncogene. The particular genotype is helpful in guiding the expected phenotype and the risk of developing MTC. Thus, it is vital that a genetic diagnosis be made in the kindred of those index patients with MTC to best guide timing for surgery and proper surveillance (4).

Care should be taken in interpreting calcitonin concentrations in infants and young children as calcitonin is normally elevated in children younger than 3 years of age (5). The definitive therapy for MTC is surgical resection prior to the tumor invading the thyroid capsule. In children with MEN 2A, if preoperative calcitonin <30 pg/mL and the tumor is sub-centimeter, then lymph node metastases is not expected. In MEN 2B, total thyroidectomy with lymph node dissection under care of a high-volume surgeon should be performed within the first few months of life with care given to preserving the parathyroid glands. In children with *de novo* mutation with MEN 2B, recognition of disease on average is made around 14 years of age by which time there is disseminated disease.

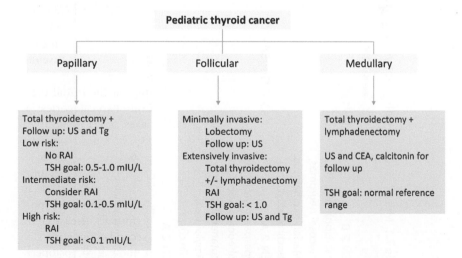

Figure 7.1 Pediatric thyroid cancer management by histology types.

Table 7.1 MEN 2 syndrome with genotype-phenotype correlation and management (4)

	Genotype	MTC risk level	Surgery	Surveillance + screening
MEN 2 B (Hirschsprung's, mucosal neuromas, Marfan-like habitus, pheochromocytoma)	M918T	HST (highest)	Total thyroidectomy <1 year; consider level VI lymph node dissection	• Examination and calcitonin, CEA q6 mo × 1 year, then q1 year • Screening for pheochromocytoma at 11 years
MEN 2 A (hyperparathyroidism, pheochromocytoma, cutaneous lichen amyloidosis, Hirschsprung's)	C634F/G/R/S/W/Y	H (high)	Total thyroidectomy <5 years of age	• Examination and calcitonin, CEA q6 mo × 1 year, then q1 year • Screening for pheochromocytoma at 11 years
MEN 2 A (hyperparathyroidism, pheochromocytoma, cutaneous lichen amyloidosis, Hirschsprung's)	All other genotypes	Mod (moderate)	Total thyroidectomy with increasing calcitonin	• Examination and calcitonin q6 mo × 1 year, then q1 year • Screening for pheochromocytoma at 16 years

If, due to local aggressive metastasis, incomplete surgery is performed, external beam radiotherapy can be considered, but overall prognosis in these patients is still poor (6) (Table 7.1).

POSTOPERATIVE MANAGEMENT OF MTC

Post-surgery, thyroid hormone should be supplemented with levothyroxine, but suppression therapy (as done in patients with PTC and FTC) is not needed. Patients should be monitored for hypocalcemia and treated with calcium and vitamin D as necessary. Surveillance management includes physical examination, neck ultrasound, TSH measurement, and calcitonin and CEA measurement.

In patients with MTC with locally advanced or disseminated disease, the goals of care and surgery should be more palliative with attention given to minimizing complications. If post-surgical calcitonin concentration is increasing significantly over 150 pg/mL, imaging studies including neck ultrasound, chest computerized tomography (CT), magnetic resonance imaging (MRI) of the liver and bone, positron emission tomography (PET) with radiotracers such as fluorodeoxyglucose ([18]FDG) or dotatate gallium (^{68}Ga-DOTATATE), and bone scintigraphy are used to localize disease. Treatment with several types of tyrosine kinase inhibitors have been studied without any definitive improvement in life expectancy (6). However, Vandetanib has been approved for treatment of pediatric advanced MTC with MEN syndrome (7). Treatment with other tyrosine kinase inhibitors should only be undertaken under a research protocol (4).

REFERENCES

1. Dermody S, Walls A, Harley EH, Jr. Pediatric Thyroid Cancer: An Update from the SEER Database 2007–2012. *Int J Pediatr Otorhinolaryngol* 2016;89:121–6.
2. Francis GL, Waguespack SG, Bauer AJ, Angelos P, Benvenga S, Cerutti JM, et al. Management Guidelines for Children with Thyroid Nodules and Differentiated Thyroid Cancer. *Thyroid* 2015;25(7):716–59.
3. Spinelli C, Rallo L, Morganti R, Mazzotti V, Inserra A, Cecchetto G, et al. Surgical Management of Follicular Thyroid Carcinoma in Children and Adolescents: A Study of 30 Cases. *J Pediatr Surg* 2019;54(3):521–6.
4. Wells SA, Jr., Asa SL, Dralle H, Elisei R, Evans DB, Gagel RF, et al. Revised American Thyroid Association Guidelines for the Management of Medullary Thyroid Carcinoma. *Thyroid* 2015;25(6):567–610.
5. Eckelt F, Vogel M, Geserick M, Kirsten T, Bae YJ, Baber R, et al. Calcitonin Measurement in Pediatrics: Reference Ranges are Gender-Dependent, Validation in Medullary Thyroid Cancer and Thyroid Diseases. *Clin Chem Lab Med* 2019;57(8):1242–50.
6. Viola D, Elisei R. Management of Medullary Thyroid Cancer. *Endocrinol Metab Clin North Am* 2019;48(1):285–301.
7. Valerio L, Pieruzzi L, Giani C, Agate L, Bottici V, Lorusso L, et al. Targeted Therapy in Thyroid Cancer: State of the Art. *Clin Oncol (R Coll Radiol).* 2017;29(5):316–324.

8

Thyroid surgery

JESSICA FAZENDIN AND BRENESSA LINDEMAN

INTRODUCTION

Surgical principles dictate that the correct operation should be performed for an appropriate indication, completed in a well-timed fashion, and be carried out with the patient's safety at the forefront of the surgeon's mind. Previous chapters in this handbook have addressed the indications for surgical intervention in the pediatric population. Here in this chapter we will provide a brief overview of thyroid surgery in the pediatric population, when key anatomic structures are encountered during surgery, and how they are handled intraoperatively. We will also describe the relatively infrequent incidence of complications as related to thyroid surgery.

THYROID ANATOMY

A surgical endocrinologist's approach to thyroid surgery must start with a thorough understanding of the gland's anatomy. The thyroid lies anterolateral to the trachea and is attached to it by the short, fibrous ligament of Berry. Typical thyroids are bi-lobed, their shape often likened to a butterfly, with a normal gland weighing between 15 and 20 g. As with other endocrine organs, the thyroid has a robust and intercalated system for arterial supply and venous drainage. The thyroid is supplied by two main arteries, and their subsequent branches. The superior thyroid artery, the first branch of the external carotid artery, supplies the superior poles of the gland, with the inferior thyroid artery, arising from the thyrocervical trunk, supplying the inferior poles. The inferior thyroid artery also supplies both upper and lower parathyroid glands. The venous drainage is three-fold via the superior, middle, and inferior thyroid veins, of which the first two drain into the internal jugular vein and the inferior vein drains into the brachio-cephalic vein. The gland has a rich lymphatic drainage system via the Delphian (pretracheal), laryngeal, paratracheal, and lateral cervical nodes. The most common site of lymphatic drainage is to the paratracheal nodes within the central compartment of the neck (2).

Fundamental to the safe completion of neck surgery is an intimate knowledge of the nerves that run alongside and near the thyroid: the recurrent and superior laryngeal nerves. The recurrent laryngeal nerve provides both motor and sensory control to the intrinsic muscles of the larynx and the glottis and larynx, respectively, while the external branch of the superior laryngeal nerve provides motor control to the cricothyroid muscle.

SURGICAL TECHNIQUE

While there have been recent innovations in the approach to thyroid surgery in the adult population, including endoscopic and minimally invasive techniques, these have not been studied or routinely utilized in the pediatric population. For the purposes of this handbook, we will focus on the traditional, open approach through the anterior neck.

Adjuncts to surgery and patient positioning

The patient lays supine or in a modified semi-Fowler's (beach chair) position on the operating table with their arms tucked at both sides and their neck in slight extension. At the discretion of the surgeon, an endotracheal tube with EMG nerve monitoring can be used to stimulate the vagus, recurrent, and superior laryngeal nerves. It should be noted that the nerve monitor is no substitute for expert, meticulous dissection, and the use of nerve monitoring has not been shown to decrease the incidence of nerve injury among experienced surgeons, except in re-operative neck surgery (3).

Incision and exposure of the thyroid

A transverse curvilinear cervical incision is made 1–2 fingerbreadths above the sternal notch and at least 1 fingerbreadth below the cricoid cartilage. Every effort is made to limit the incision to 3–5 cm in length; however, this is dependent on the size of the gland and the extent of surgery to be performed. Care is taken to hide the incision within a natural crease within the skin. The incision is carried down through the skin, subcutaneous tissue, and platysma transversely, and skin flaps are raised superiorly and inferiorly in the sub-platysmal plane. Care is taken to separate the anterior jugular veins from the flaps, allowing them to remain lying on the strap muscles. The sternohyoid and sternothyroid muscles are then divided in the midline and the sternothyroid fibers lifted off of the thyroid parenchyma. At this point, if a nerve monitor is utilized, a signal from the vagus nerve can be obtained to test that the circuit is intact prior to initiation of dissection in the paratracheal space. As the paratracheal space is developed, the middle thyroid vein is routinely encountered, ligated, and divided (Figure 8.1).

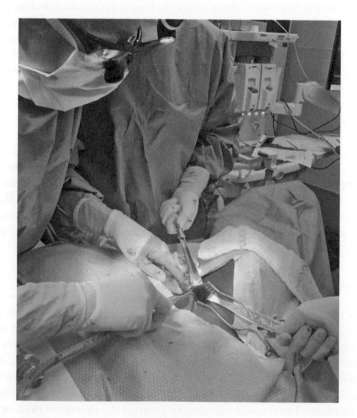

Figure 8.1 Surgical exposure of the thyroid gland.

Mobilization of thyroid

Attention is routinely first turned to the superior portion of the thyroid lobe where the superior thyroid artery both supplies the gland and tethers it to its position high in the neck. A variety of energy devices (Harmonic© [Ethicon, Sommerville, NJ], Ligasure© [Covidien, Minneapolis, MN]), surgical clips, or manual sutures can be used to ligate the vessels and separate them from the thyroid. Care must be taken at this step to preserve the external branch of the superior laryngeal nerve, which typically runs along the lateral musculature of the larynx, by maintaining dissection right on the thyroid capsule itself. Once the superior pole has been freed, the thyroid lobe is then rotated anteriorly and medially to identify the critical structures lying along its posterior surface.

Identification of the RLN

Once the thyroid is mobilized, identification of the recurrent laryngeal nerve must be made in order to reduce the incidence of injury. Its course is most often parallel to the trachea within the tracheoesophageal groove and in close proximity to the branches of the inferior thyroid artery. If utilized, a nerve monitor can confirm that the nerve has maintained its function following the surgeon's careful dissection and visual identification of the nerve. The RLN should be traced superiorly, once identified, until it makes a characteristic turn before it enters the larynx.

Preservation of the parathryroids

During mobilization of the thyroid, care must be made to preserve each of the four parathyroid glands. This can be accomplished by careful dissection of the medial aspect of each parathyroid gland to release its capsular attachments from its seat on the thyroid, gently sweeping it laterally on a vascular pedicle. If a gland is inadvertently devascularized during this step, it should be removed and placed on cold, sterile saline in preparation for re-implantation within the strap muscles or sternocleidomastoid muscle of the neck.

Removal of thyroid

Now that the surgeon is assured of the preservation of the parathyroid glands and the course of the RLN, the inferior thyroid artery can be dissected and divided, as the superior thyroid artery was earlier (Figure 8.2). To avoid injury to the aforementioned structures, this is accomplished as close to the thyroid capsule as possible, dividing all small branches with an energy device, clips, or suture. The gland can then be separated from the trachea by isolating the gland from Berry's ligament. The surgeon can elect to transect the thyroid at the level of the isthmus to complete a thyroid lobectomy, or repeat the previously described steps on the contralateral side if a total thyroidectomy is indicated. Once the specimen

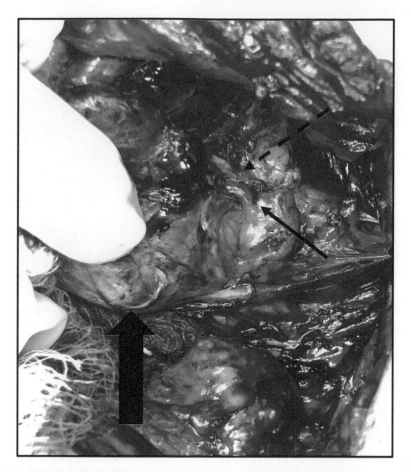

Figure 8.2 Intraoperative anatomy during thyroidectomy. The thick arrow shows the thyroid gland reflected medially. The solid arrow shows a preserved parathyroid gland. The dashed arrow points to the recurrent laryngeal nerve, carefully dissected away from the thyroid lobe.

is removed, it is crucial to inspect the surgical bed for meticulous hemostasis. If a nerve monitor was used, an exit signal obtained from the vagus nerve could then be obtained to ensure that the nerve was not injured at any point in the course of the dissection.

Closure

The strap muscles are approximated in the midline and closed with absorbable suture. Many surgeons elect to leave a gap at the inferior aspect of the strap muscles to decompress the paratracheal space if a hematoma should form postoperatively. The platysma is then closed transversely, also with absorbable suture. The

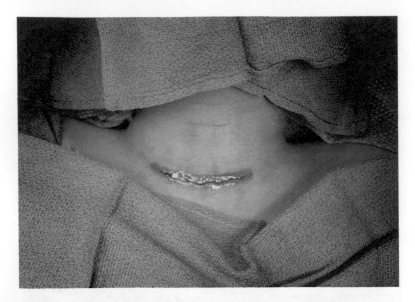

Figure 8.3 Transverse cervical incision, placed within a neck fold, at the conclusion of a thyroidectomy.

skin is then closed with a subcutaneous stitch before it is covered with surgical glue (Dermabond©, Ethicon, Somerville, NJ) or steri-strips (Figure 8.3).

RECOVERY

Thyroid surgery can be performed safely in most cases on an outpatient basis. Our practice is to obtain a parathyroid hormone level in the recovery room after total thyroidectomy to help predict temporary hypocalcemia. If this level is low, we prescribe oral calcium carbonate tablets (Tums©) with or without calcitriol. Calcium and PTH levels are then checked 2 weeks after surgery.

Pediatric patients may experience sore throat from the placement of the endotracheal tube. Ibuprofen and/or acetaminophen alone are usually sufficient for pain control. There are no stitches to remove, and there are very few activity restrictions placed on children, allowing them to return to school within days postoperatively.

Thyroid hormone replacement is normally started on the first postoperative day after total thyroidectomy (Figure 8.4). A TSH is then checked at the 2-week postoperative visit and again at 6 weeks.

COMPLICATIONS

As described in the "Surgical technique" section, extreme care is taken to preserve the nerves within the neck during thyroid surgery. If the superior laryngeal nerve is injured, patients can experience alterations in voice pitch and occasional difficulties swallowing. If the RLN is injured on one side, patients will typically

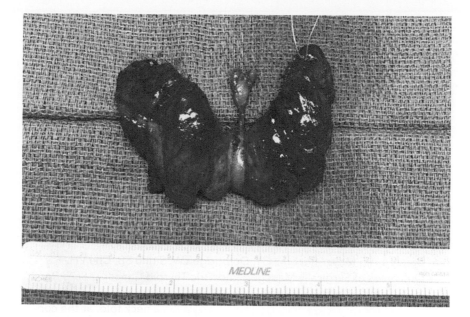

Figure 8.4 Total thyroid specimen containing the right and left lobes, the thyroid isthmus, and the pyramidal lobe in the center. Stitch marks the upper pole of the left lobe.

exhibit a hoarse or whisper-like voice that recovers in weeks to months in most cases. If both RLNs are injured, the patient could experience both vocal cords frozen in apposition to one another, creating an airway emergency necessitating temporary tracheostomy. In a recent high-volume, pediatric single-institution study, incidence of temporary hoarseness and permanent hoarseness was 1.9% and 0.4% respectively. Temporary hypocalcemia, reported as high as 7.9%, can also be experienced if there is stunning to the parathyroids during removal of the thyroid, with a small percentage of individuals experiencing permanent hypocalcemia. This can happen more frequently in younger patients, those with hyperthyroidism, and more extensive dissection as in lymphadenectomy procedures. In a minority of patients (1.3%), return to the operating room for hematoma evacuation is required (4). Thankfully, these complications have a very low incidence, and pediatric thyroid surgery has been shown to have excellent outcomes in the absence of long-term negative sequelae in the hands of an experienced, high-volume surgeon (5, 6).

REFERENCES

1. Al-Qurayshi Z, Robins R, Hauch A, Randolph GW, Kandil E. Association of Surgeon Volume with Outcomes and Cost Savings Following Thyroidectomy: A National Forecast. *JAMA Otolaryngol Head Neck Surg* 2016;142(1):32–9.

2. McMullen TPW, Delbridge LW. Thyroid Embryology, Anatomy, and Physiology: A Review for the Surgeon. In: Hubbard JGH, Inabnet WB, Lo CY, et al. editors. *Endocrine Surgery: Principles and Practice*. London: Springer-Verlag; 2011: 3–16.
3. Barcynski M, Konturek A, Pragacz K, Papeier A, Stopa M, Nowak W. Intraoperative Nerve Monitoring Can Reduce Prevalence of Recurrent Laryngeal Nerve Injury in Thyroid Reoperations: Results of A Retrospective Cohort Study. *World J Surg* 2014;38(3):599–606.
4. Baumgarten HD, Bauer AJ, Isaza A, Mostoufi-Moab S, Kazahay K, Adzick NS. Surgical Management of Pediatric Thyroid Disease: Complication Rates after Thryoidectomy at the Children's Hospital of Philadelphia High-Volume Pediatric Thyroid Center. *J Ped Surg* Oct 2019;54(10):1969–75.
5. Burke JF, Sippel RS, Chen H. Evolution of Pediatric Thyroid Surgery at a Tertiary Medical Center. *J Surg Res* 2012 Oct;177(2):268–74.
6. Bargren AE, Meyer-Rochow GY, Delbridge LW, Sidhu SB, Chen H. Outcomes of Surgically Managed Pediatric Thyroid Cancer. *J Surg Res* 2009 Sep;156(1):70–3.

9

Laboratory evaluation of parathyroid gland function

ALLEN W. ROOT

Parathyroid hormone (PTH) is an essential component of the system that regulates calcium and phosphate homeostasis that is maintained by the interaction of PTH and the primary bioactive metabolite of vitamin D—1,25-dihydroxyvitamin D (calcitriol)—acting upon the absorption of these ions in the small intestine, the proximal renal tubular reabsorption of filtered calcium and its excretion of phosphate, the deposition of these analytes into bone by the osteoblast, and their reabsorption from this site by the osteoclast (Figures 9.1, 9.2) (1). Calcitonin, a product of the parafollicular "C" cells of the thyroid gland that lowers serum calcium concentrations by impairing its release from bone and increasing its urinary excretion, plays a minor role in this regulatory process. Forty percent of the total serum calcium concentration is bound to albumin and globulin, 10–15% is linked to citrate, phosphate, lactate, bicarbonate, and sulfate, and 45–50% is biologically active free or ionized calcium (Ca^{2+}). Alterations in blood pH alter the distribution of calcium and thus modulate the concentration of Ca^{2+} as the binding of Ca^{2+} to albumin declines with acidosis and increases with alkalosis. Circulating Ca^{2+} is detected by the calcium-sensing receptor (CaSR), encoded by *CASR*, a guanosine triphosphate-coupled seven transmembrane receptor expressed on the cell membrane of the PTH-secreting chief cells of the parathyroid glands, epithelial cells of the renal tubules, and osteoblasts. When the Ca^{2+} concentration declines, CaSR signaling in the parathyroid glands activates the intracellular phosphatidylinositol 4,5 bisphosphate signal transduction pathway leading to rapid release of Ca^{2+} from intracellular storage sites followed by increase in synthesis and secretion of PTH. In response to increasing serum concentrations of Ca^{2+}, the parafollicular cells of the thyroid gland synthesize calcitonin which suppresses osteoclast-mediated resorption of bone, thereby lowering serum calcium values. Optimally, Ca^{2+} concentrations should be determined in

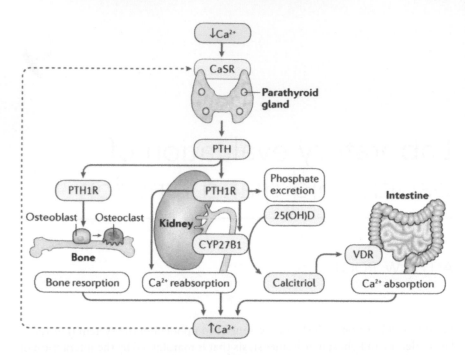

Figure 9.1 Regulation of calcium homeostasis. Parathyroid hormone (PTH) and calcitriol (1,25[OH]$_2$D$_3$) stimulate the absorption of calcium (Ca^{2+}) from the small intestine, renal tubule, and bone. The Ca^{2+}-sensing receptor (CaSR) modulates Ca^{2+} mediated activity of the parathyroid glands and the renal tubules. Renal tubular generation of calcitriol is stimulated by both hypocalcemia and hypophosphatemia, and calcitriol increases intestinal absorption of calcium and phosphate. PTH increases the renal tubular reabsorption of calcium while inhibiting renal tubular reabsorption of phosphate. Increasing serum concentrations of calcium inhibit secretion of PTH. (Fibroblast growth factor-23 [FGF23], a phosphatonin secreted by osteoblasts and osteocytes, inhibits renal tubular reabsorption of phosphate and synthesis of calcitriol. Calcitonin, a product of the thyroid gland C cells, inhibits resorption of calcium from bone.) (Reproduced from [9] with permission.)

serum specimens collected without a tourniquet from a calm, fasting patient and with a normal respiratory rate in tubes containing a gel separator (2). When necessary, the Ca^{2+} concentration may be determined in specimens collected in tubes containing lithium/heparin. Ca^{2+} is measured by an ion-selective electrode. Serum concentrations of calcium are high *in utero* and at birth and decline in the first 24 hours after delivery. In children older than 1 year of age, the total calcium concentration (mg/dL) varies by age: 1–5 years: 9.4–10.8; 6–12 years: 9.4–10.2; >20 years: 8.8–10.2. Ca^{2+} values (mg/dL) are: 1 month: 5.2–6.1; 3 months: 5.2–6.0; 12 months: 5.0–5.6; in older children Ca^{2+} values range between 4.8 and 5.3 (1.20–1.40 mmol/L). Total calcium levels are low in the hypoproteinemic/hypoalbuminemic patient—a correction for hypoalbuminemia may be calculated by

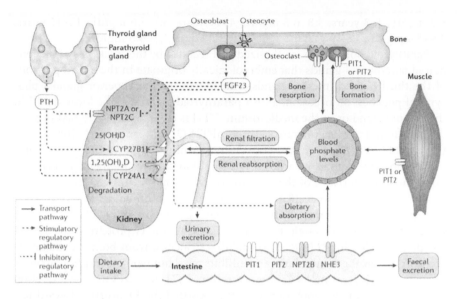

Figure 9.2 Regulation of phosphate homeostasis. After ingestion, phosphate is absorbed from the gastrointestinal tract both passively by paracellular mechanisms and through active phosphate co-transporters (NP2B, NHE3, PIT1, PIT2). Parathyroid hormone (PTH) and fibroblast growth factor 23 (FGF23) decease serum concentrations of phosphate by increasing its urinary excretion by decreasing renal tubular expression of phosphate co-transporter proteins (NPT2A, NPT2C). FGF23 is synthesized by osteoblasts and osteocytes; its production is decreased by low serum phosphate levels and by PHEX (phosphate regulating gene with homologies to endopeptidases on the X chromosome), dentin matrix protein 1 (DMP1), and ectonucleotide pyrophosphate/phosphodiesterase 1 (ENPP1), all three of which agents are also synthesized by bone cells. PTH increases while FGF23 depresses the synthesis of calcitriol (1,25 dihydroxyvitamin D). (Reproduced from [10], with permission.)

adding 0.8 mg/dL to the recorded total calcium concentration for every decrease in albumin concentration of 1 g/dL; however, the agreement between calculated and measured Ca^{2+} concentrations is limited (2).

Phosphate is second to calcium in abundance; this anion is present in DNA and RNA nucleotides, essential for the generation of energy as adenosine triphosphate (ATP), and a component of cell membranes, signal transduction pathways, and the bone mineral—hydroxyapatite. It is absorbed by the intestinal duodenum and jejunum, filtered through the renal glomerulus to be reabsorbed by the proximal renal tubule or excreted in urine, and deposited into bone linked to calcium as hydroxyapatite from which site it may be reabsorbed by PTH and calcitriol. Under usual circumstances, the serum concentrations of calcium and phosphate are reciprocally related, and the calcium × phosphate product approximates 30. Serum concentrations of phosphate decrease with age: between 0 and 5 days serum phosphate levels range between 4.8 and

8.2 mg/dL; 1–3 years: 3.8–6.5 mg/dL; 4–11 years: 3.7–5.6 mg/dL; 12–15 years: 2.9–5.4 mg/dL; 16–19 years: 2.7–4.7 mg/dL; adult: 2.5–4.5 mg/dL.

Parathyroid hormone is synthesized and secreted by the chief cells of the four paired parathyroid glands that embryologically originate in the dorsal portions of the third (paired inferior glands) and fourth (paired superior glands) pharyngeal pouches; on occasion, a fifth parathyroid gland may be located within the thyroid gland or in the mediastinum. PTH is an 84 amino acid (aa) peptide derived from its 115 aa precursor—preproPTH (3). In serum PTH circulates in the intact bioactive 84 aa form, as an amino terminal fragment that may or may not be bioactive, and as a carboxyl terminal bioinactive fragment. Depending upon the characteristics of the immunoassay, normal serum concentrations of intact PTH range between 10 and 55 pg/mL, amino terminal PTH 8 and 24 pg/mL, and carboxyl terminal PTH 50 and 330 pg/mL. The intracellular signal of PTH is transmitted through its seven transmembrane G-protein coupled PTH receptor encoded by *PTH1R*. PTH mobilizes calcium from bone, facilitates its reabsorption by the renal tubule, and inhibits renal tubular reabsorption of phosphate thereby increasing its urinary excretion. PTH increases urinary excretion of cyclic adenosine monophosphate (cyclic AMP). (The Ellsworth–Howard test employs biosynthetic PTH$^{1-34}$ to determine renal tubular responsiveness to PTH: the urinary excretion of phosphate and cyclic AMP increase after administration of PTH$^{1-34}$ to the subject with intact renal tubular function.) PTH stimulates synthesis of the bioactive metabolite of vitamin D (calcitriol) (*vide infra*). Parathyroid hormone-like hormone (PTHLH) is a 141 aa peptide whose activity is also mediated by the PTH1R that has many biologic activities in common with PTH; serum concentrations of PTHrP are usually <2 pmol/L. When enlarged, the parathyroid glands may be visualized by ultrasonography, technetium^{99m}-labeled sestamibi scintigraphy with/without co-administration of iodine^{123}, computed tomography (CT), and magnetic resonance imaging (MRI). Hybrid technologies for visualization of the enlarged parathyroid gland include ^{11}C-methionine positron-emission tomography (PET), ^{11}C-choline PET/CT, and 3-tesla simultaneous PET/MRI (4, 5). Intraoperative identification of PTH-secreting parathyroid tissue may be accomplished by serial measurements of serum PTH concentrations before and after removal of the suspicious mass, an expensive and time-consuming procedure, and near-infrared autofluorescence possibly with superimposition of the image upon the surgical field of vision (6).

Calcitonin is a 32 aa product of the thyroid parafollicular or "C" cell that impairs reabsorption of skeletal calcium and phosphate and increases urinary excretion of calcium. It functions through binding to its 7-transmembrane, G-protein coupled receptor (encoded by *CALCA*). As serum Ca^{2+} concentrations increase, calcitonin is secreted by thyroid C cells. Normal calcitonin concentrations are highest in neonates (<34 pg/mL at 1 month of age) and decline thereafter (children and adults <14 pg/mL).

Vitamin D may be produced by skin upon exposure to ultraviolet B light (cholecalciferol—vitamin D$_3$) or ingested as plant- or animal-based ergocalciferol (vitamin D_2). Vitamin D_3 must be hydroxylated at carbon-25 in the liver (forming 25-hydroxyvitamin D_3 = calcidiol) and then at carbon-1 in the renal tubule in order to produce bioactive 1,25 dihydroxyvitamin D_3 (calcitriol) that acts through a nuclear vitamin D receptor in association with the retinoic acid receptor to modulate expression of target genes. Serum concentrations of calcidiol reflect body stores of this vitamin; current recommendations for interpretation of the serum calcidiol concentration are deficiency of vitamin D: <12 ng/mL; insufficiency: 12–20 ng/mL; sufficiency: >20–50 ng/mL; toxicity: >100 ng/mL if associated with hypercalcemia.

Fibroblast growth factor-23 (FGF23) is a phosphatonin, a protein that impairs renal tubular reabsorption of phosphate, decreases renal synthesis of calcitriol and thereby depresses intestinal absorption of calcium and phosphate, and increases the synthesis and urinary excretion of water-soluble 1,24,25-trihydroxyvitamin D (9). FGF23 is expressed primarily by osteoblasts and osteocytes. FGF23 links to the "c" isoform of tyrosine kinase FGF receptors (FGFR) 1, 2, and 3. FGF23 binds to the dimeric co-receptor three-member complex—αKlotho/FGFR1(IIIc)/heparan sulfate—and depresses renal tubular reabsorption of phosphate, intestinal absorption of phosphate, synthesis of calcitriol, and secretion of PTH. Normal serum concentrations of FGF23 range between 5 and 210 U/mL and are increased in subjects with hypophosphatemia of diverse pathogenesis.

After careful historical review and physical examinations, the evaluation of disorders of calcium homeostasis begins with measurements of serum concentrations of total calcium and Ca^{2+}, phosphate, creatinine, and intact PTH[1-84] (7). Depending upon whether the problem one is attempting to solve is associated with hypocalcemia, hypercalcemia, or eucalcemia, further evaluation is undertaken. Thus, in the absence of intestinal malabsorption or severe compromise of renal function, the hypocalcemic, hyperphosphatemic child with reproducibly low or unmeasurable serum PTH concentrations most likely has hypoparathyroidism—prompting a search for the cause of parathyroid gland dysfunction such as congenital aplasia or hypoplasia of the parathyroid glands (e.g., the DiGeorge syndrome due to aberrant differentiation of structures derived from the third and fourth branchial pouches; variants of GATA3, NEBL, TBCE, and CHD7 may also be associated with abnormal differentiation of the parathyroid glands, while variants of PTH may result in abnormal synthesis of its product), a destructive autoimmune process affecting the parathyroid glands (isolated or associated with autoimmune polyendocrine syndrome type 1 related to a variant of AIRE), or a post-cervical surgical insult. Gain-of-function variants of CASR, the gene encoding the calcium-sensing receptor, are also associated with suppressed synthesis/secretion of PTH and resultant hypocalcemia. If serum PTH concentrations are elevated in the hypocalcemic, hyperphosphatemic patient, then abnormalities of PTH function (pseudohypoparathyroidism) should be evaluated including those due to variants of GNAS1 encoding the alpha subunit of the guanine nucleotide binding protein. In the hypocalcemic subject with elevated serum concentrations of PTH but normal or low serum levels of phosphate, intestinal absorption of calcium may be extremely low due to decreased intake of this cation or its impaired intestinal absorption due to vitamin D deficiency (identified by subnormal serum concentrations of calcidiol) or an abnormality of vitamin D metabolism and the production of calcitriol. Severe renal impairment may also hinder the synthesis of calcitriol. In the presence of high serum levels of calcitriol, an abnormality of the vitamin D receptor should be considered. Deficiency of magnesium stores may be associated with subnormal secretion of PTH and consequent hypocalcemia. Please see Table 9.1 for an evaluation of a hypocalcemic child, correlating laboratory findings with clinical conditions.

Hypercalcemia may develop because of increased synthesis and secretion of PTH, excessive intake of vitamin D, calcium, or medications, sudden immobilization of the normally active adolescent, or in association with concurrent disease (hyperthyroidism, hypoadrenocorticism, pheochromocytoma) (8). Thus, hyperparathyroidism may be primary and sporadic, familial and isolated or associated with the syndromes of multiple endocrine neoplasia types 1 and 2, or related to loss-of-function variants of *CASR* or to inhibitory autoantibodies directed to CaSR. The synthesis of PTHrP may be increased in subjects with a neoplasm. Vitamin D intoxication and chronic granulomatous diseases result in increased synthesis of calcitriol leading to hyperabsorption of intestinal calcium and hypercalcemia. Several medications (lithium, thiazide diuretics, vitamin A) also can cause hypercalcemia, in part by increasing the rate of bone resorption. See Table 9.2 for an evaluation of a hypercalcemic child correlating laboratory findings with clinical conditions.

Table 9.1 Evaluation of hypocalcemic ($\downarrow$Ca^{2+}) child

Laboratory findings	Condition
$\uparrow$PO$_4$-, normal creatinine, $\downarrow$PTH	Hypoparathyroidism: • Dysmorphic features: DiGeorge syndrome • Gene variants (PTH, GATA3, TBCE, CHD7, GCM2, CASR, FAM111A) • Autoimmune disorder (isolated or APS1) • Surgical insult
$\downarrow$Mg^{2+}	Hypomagnesemia
$\uparrow$PTH	Pseudohypoparathyroidism (*GNAS1*, *STX16*)
$\uparrow$Creatinine	Chronic renal disease
$\downarrow$Total protein	Hypoproteinemia
$\downarrow$PO$_4$-, $\downarrow$25-hydroxyvitamin D	Vitamin D deficiency

Ca^{2+}: calcium, PO$_4$-: phosphate, PTH: parathyroid hormone, APS1: autoimmune polyglandular syndrome type 1.

Table 9.2 Evaluation of hypercalcemic ($\uparrow Ca^{2+}$) child

Laboratory findings	Condition
$\downarrow PO_{4-}$, normal creatinine, $\uparrow PTH$	Hyperparathyroidism:
	• Adenoma (MEN1, CDC73)
	• Ectopic parathyroid gland
	• Hyperplastic parathyroid glands
$\downarrow PTH$	• Familial benign hypercalcemia (*CASR, GNA11, AP2S1*)
	• Williams syndrome (del17q11.23)
	• Immobilization syndrome
	• Milk-alkali syndrome
$\uparrow PTHrP$	Neoplasia
$\uparrow$Total protein	Hyperproteinemia
$\uparrow PO_{4-}$, $\uparrow$25-hydroxyvitamin D, $\uparrow$1,25-dihydroxyvitamin D	• Vitamin D excess
	• Granulomatous disease (e.g., sarcoidosis)

Ca^{2+}: calcium, PO_{4-}: phosphate, PTH: parathyroid hormone, MEN: multiple endocrine neoplasia.

REFERENCES

1. Root AW. Disorders of Mineral Metabolism. In: Sperling M, editor. *Pediatric Endocrinology*. 5th ed. 2019, Elsevier.
2. Jafri L, Khan AH, Azeem S. Ionized Calcium Measurement in Serum and Plasma by Ion Selective Electrodes: Comparison of Measured and Calculated Parameters. *Indian J Clin Biochem* 2014;29(3):327–32.
3. Wiren KM, Potts JT, Jr., Kronenberg HM. Importance of the Propeptide Sequence of Human Preproparathyroid Hormone for Signal Sequence Function. *J Biol Chem* 1988;263(36):19771–7.
4. Parvinian A, Martin-Macintosh EL, Goenka AH, Durski JM, Mullan BP, Kemp BJ, et al. (11). 11C-choline PET/CT for Detection and Localization of Parathyroid Adenomas. *AJR Am J Roentgenol* 2018;210(2):418–22.
5. Purz S, Kluge R, Barthel H, Steinert F, Stumpp P, Kahn T, Sabri O. Visualization of Ectopic Parathyroid Adenomas. *N Engl J Med* 2013;369(21):2067–9.
6. McWade MA, Thomas G, Nguyen JQ, Sanders ME, Solorzano CC, Mahadevan-Jansen A. Enhancing Parathyroid Gland Visualization Using a Near Infrared Fluorescence-Based Overlay Imaging System. *J Am Coll Surg* 2019;228(5):730–43.
7. Carpenter T. Etiology of Hypocalcemia in Infants and Children. *Uptodate.* 2019;2019:1–30.
8. Shane E. Etiology of Hypercalcemia. *Uptodate.* 2019:1–14.

9. Mannstadt M, Bilezikian JP, Thakker RV, Hannan FM, Clarke BL, Rejnmark L, et al. Hypoparathyroidism. *Nat Rev Dis Primers* 2017;3(1):17080.
10. Minisola S, Peacock M, Fukumoto S, Cipriani C, Pepe J, Tella SH, Collins MT. Tumour-Induced Osteomalacia. *Nat Rev Dis Primers* 2017;3:17044.

10

Imaging of the parathyroid gland

SOPHIE DREAM AND TRACY S. WANG

INTRODUCTION

Primary hyperparathyroidism (pHPT) in the pediatric population is rare, with an incidence of 2–5 per 100,000 (1). For many years, bilateral exploration of all four parathyroid glands has been the gold standard for patients undergoing parathyroidectomy for pHPT. However, for the majority of both adult and pediatric patients with pHPT, the etiology is secondary to a single adenoma (2). Therefore, the role of preoperative imaging for patients with pHPT has come to aid in the surgical approach to parathyroid disease; namely, if a single enlarged parathyroid adenoma is identified on preoperative imaging, a minimally invasive (focused) approach to parathyroidectomy is appropriate when an intraoperative adjunct, such as intraoperative parathyroid hormone (PTH) monitoring, is used to confirm adequate resection (3, 4).

The judicious use of imaging should be maintained for preoperative localization, keeping in mind that diagnosis and the decision to proceed with surgery are based on biochemical evaluation and patient factors. Per the 2016 American Association of Endocrine Surgeons (AAES) Guidelines for the Definitive Management of Primary Hyperparathyroidism, patients who are deemed candidates for parathyroidectomy should undergo imaging at the recommendation of an expert clinician who is familiar with regional imaging capabilities, as this may increase localization sensitivity up to 92% (3). Preoperative imaging is utilized for operative planning; a negative imaging study does not preclude parathyroidectomy (3). Additionally, imaging is known to be significantly less accurate in patients with multi-gland disease (MGD) (5). Patients known to have or at high risk for MGD should not routinely undergo minimally invasive parathyroidectomy, but should, at minimum, have preoperative thyroid ultrasound to rule out contaminate thyroid pathology (3). This is particularly important in the pediatric population when, given patient age, there is a high suspicion for MGD and routine referral for genetic counseling also is recommended.

This chapter provides an overview of parathyroid imaging options. Given the paucity of literature examining the utility of parathyroid imaging in children, the information provided is primarily based on literature from adult populations with consideration of pediatric patients.

ULTRASOUND

The accessibility and ease of ultrasound (US) make it a widely utilized first choice for an imaging modality for the localization of a parathyroid adenoma (4). On US imaging, the normal parathyroid gland is not detected, given its small size. However, abnormal parathyroid glands can appear as hypoechoic, round, solid masses adjacent to the thyroid gland. In the eutopic location, an abnormal parathyroid gland can be detected adjected or posterior to the upper or lower thyroid poles. Doppler US may demonstrate a feeding artery to the gland (Figure 10.1). Enlarged parathyroid glands will additionally have a hyperechoic ventral line where the gland is separated from the thyroid gland by its capsule, which may help to distinguish an abnormal parathyroid within the thyroid from an adenomatous thyroid nodule (6).

The role of US in patients with pHPT additionally serves to evaluate the thyroid gland for abnormalities. Approximately 25–50% of patients with pHPT will have concomitant thyroid pathology that should be evaluated prior to planned parathyroidectomy, as 4–6% of patients may have a concurrent thyroid malignancy (7–9). Complete preoperative work-up of concurrent thyroid pathology prevents future reoperation that places patients at an increased risk of complications, such as hypoparathyroidism and recurrent laryngeal nerve injury (3). Additionally, complete preoperative work-up of thyroid nodules may significantly decrease the rate of unnecessary thyroid resection for incidentally found thyroid nodules discovered intraoperatively in patients undergoing parathyroidectomy (10). Recommendations for fine needle aspiration biopsy of thyroid nodules should follow current recommendations in the thyroid literature (11–14).

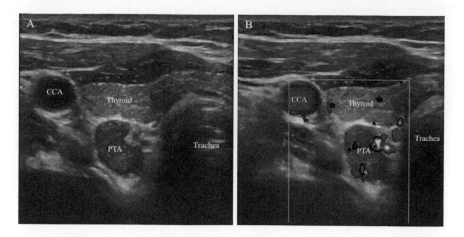

Figure 10.1 Right transverse parathyroid ultrasound with right parathyroid adenoma (A) demonstrating polar vascularity (B) on color flow. (CCA—common carotid artery; PTA—parathyroid adenoma.)

While parathyroid US has a relatively low cost, is readily accessible, and does not expose patients to ionizing radiation, it has several disadvantages (15). One of these is the wide operator-dependent variability, with sensitivities ranging from 57 to 89% for solitary adenomas, with surgeon-performed ultrasound having a reported sensitivity of 76% (16–18). Additionally, parathyroid glands located in the retrotracheal and retroesophageal spaces are usually not visible secondary to their depth and the inability of ultrasound to transmit through gas-containing structures. Glands within the mediastinum are also not detected on US imaging, as overlaying bone obscures ultrasound images.

Intrathyroidal parathyroid glands are difficult to distinguish from thyroid nodules, as they appear as round, solid, and hypoechoic mass within the thyroid with US. Incidentally biopsied parathyroid adenomas within the thyroid gland on pathology appear similar to follicular thyroid lesions on cytology, but may be distinguished using a PTH washout. Fine needle aspiration biopsy (FNAB) of parathyroid glands, however, is not advised as it may result in seeding of parathyroid tissue, resulting in parathyromatosis in benign disease and dissemination of malignant lesions (3, 19). Additionally, FNAB of parathyroid glands results in scarring that may complicate surgery and results in histological alterations on pathology that are concerning for parathyroid cancer (3, 20–22).

PARATHYROID SCINTIGRAPHY

The use of parathyroid scintigraphy began in the 1980s, with gradual evolution of the technique over time. This evolution has led to multiple techniques, with variation in the type of radiopharmaceutical administered, isotope dosing, and image-acquisition protocols (23).

Planar imaging

The most common planar method, dual-phase single-isotope imaging, utilizes a single isotope, ^{99m}Tc sestamibi, over time to obtain multiple imaging phases. In dual-phase single-isotope imaging patients receive an intravenous injection of ^{99m}Tc sestamibi, which is concentrated intracellularly in mitochondria. An initial image is performed at 10–15 minutes and then again after 90 minutes to 3 hours. In the early phase, ^{99m}Tc sestamibi distributes to the parotid, submandibular, salivary glands, thyroid gland, heart, and liver. The prominence of mitochondria-rich oxyphil cells, parathyroid adenomas, and hyperplasic parathyroid glands result in retained ^{99m}Tc sestamibi. Due to the more rapid washout of ^{99m}Tc sestamibi from the thyroid gland than hyperfunctioning parathyroid glands, delayed imaging may identify abnormal parathyroid glands (Figure 10.2).

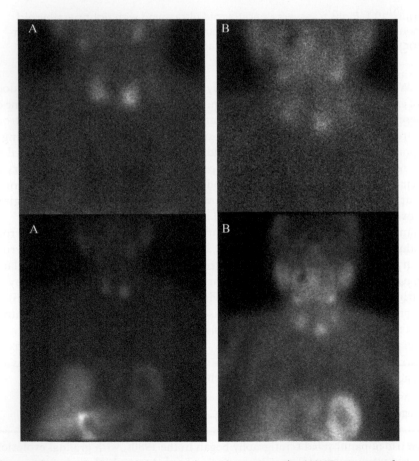

Figure 10.2 Dual-phase planar parathyroid scintigraphy (A) 15 minutes after ^{99m}Tc sestamibi injection and (B) 2-hour delayed image consistent with left parathyroid adenoma.

Another method for planar parathyroid scintigraphy is single-phase dual-isotope subtraction. With this technique, an initial image is obtained using ^{99m}Tc sestamibi to visualize hyperfunctioning parathyroid glands and the thyroid gland. An additional image is obtained with a second isotope, ^{123}I or ^{99m}Tc pertechnetate, which only visualizes the thyroid gland. The two images are digitally subtracted from each other; the remaining radioactivity represents any hyperfunctioning parathyroid gland. To minimize artifact, the two sets of images must be identical, requiring the patient to be immobile for a longer period of time.

Neither method, dual-phase single-isotope nor single-phase dual-isotope subtraction imaging, has proven to be superior; however, single-isotope dual-phase imaging is the most widely performed today due to fewer technical challenges and improved image quality (24, 25). Planar imaging has wide variability in the ability to detect a parathyroid adenoma with sensitivities ranging from 34 to 74% (26–28).

Single photon emission tomography (SPECT)

The utility of three-dimensional scintigraphy with SPECT has improved the sensitivity and localization of hyperfunctioning parathyroid glands, ranging from 67 to 73% (27, 29). SPECT images are performed in an axial fashion and are obtained using a dual-detector gamma camera system. Images are acquired in early and delayed timing similar to planar ^{99m}Tc sestamibi scanning. On SPECT imaging, hyperfunctioning parathyroid glands will accumulate more radiotracer than the thyroid gland. A hyperfunctioning parathyroid gland may have delayed washout when compared to thyroid, with retained radiotracer. A CT scan may also be obtained with SPECT imaging to allow improved anatomic definition; these images may be fused (SPECT/CT) (23) (Figure 10.3). When compared to SPECT, SPECT/CT has been shown to have higher sensitivity ranging from 77 to 94% (28–30).

A meta-analysis performed by Wong et al. evaluated the utility of parathyroid scintigraphy; they demonstrated an incremental increase in imaging ability to localize a parathyroid adenoma from planar imaging, SPECT imaging, and SPECT/CT, with overall sensitivities of 70%, 74%, and 86%, respectively (28).

FOUR-DIMENSIONAL CT SCAN

Four-dimensional (4D)-CT is a relatively new imaging modality for parathyroid disease that involves cross-sectional axial imaging with sagittal and coronal reformats with contrasted phases that extend from the angle of the mandible to the carina. The fourth dimension in this study is contrast enhancement overtime. Imaging includes a non-contrast-enhanced phase, an arterial phase, and a delayed venous phase (31). In the non-contrast enhanced phase, the parathyroid gland has lower attenuation than the thyroid gland. Due to their hypervascularity, abnormal parathyroids have rapid enhancement of contrast in the arterial

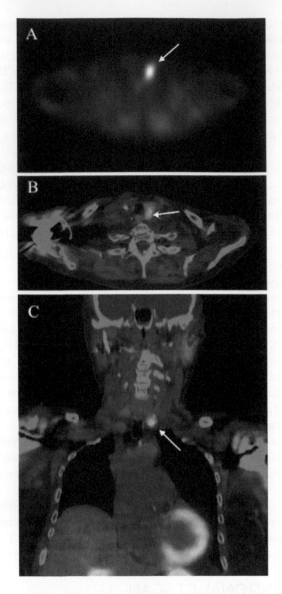

Figure 10.3 (A) Axial SPECT images, (B) axial SPECT/CT, and (C) coronal SPECT/CT with retained radiotracer uptake adjacent to the inferior left thyroid pole consistent with left parathyroid adenoma.

phase and rapid washout in the venous phase. This helps further elucidate the parathyroid gland as it will have the highest attenuation in the arterial phase and may have an identifiable polar vessel (Figure 10.4). In contrast to an abnormal parathyroid, lymph nodes have less enhancement and retain contrast through each phase. An advantage that 4D-CT presents over US and sestamibi scanning

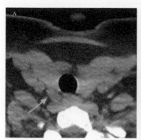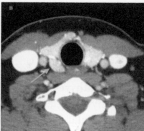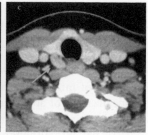

Figure 10.4 (A) Axial non-contrast phase, (B) axial early contrast phase, (C) axial delayed contrast phase. Images demonstrate early enhancing parathyroid nodule in the tracheoesophageal groove with polar vessel and rapid washout on the delayed contrast phase.

is improved sensitivity when identifying the precise location of an enlarged parathyroid utilizing the Perrier nomenclature (18, 32).

In a meta-analysis of preoperative four-dimensional CT for preoperative localization, Kluijfhout et al. estimated the sensitivity of 4D-CT to detect a parathyroid adenoma to the correct quadrant to 73% (range 48–92%), with lateralization to the correct size being 81% (33). It is notable that large-volume centers that routinely utilize 4D-CT for preoperative localization have reported localization with 93.7% accuracy for lateralization and 86.6% accuracy for quadrant (34). When compared to SPECT/CT, 4D CT provides superior preoperative localization (18, 35). The utility of four-dimensional CT is somewhat debated, with some institutions utilizing it as the initial study of choice and others using it when ultrasound and scintigraphy are inconclusive or in the re-operative setting (4).

It is important to consider the risk of radiation exposure in the pediatric population. Hunter et al. estimated an additional annual cancer risk of 0.019% utilizing a four-phased CT scan (precontrast, immediate, early delayed, and late delayed) (34). Additional studies estimate a 20-year-old female to have a 0.1% 4D-CT-related risk of thyroid cancer, with the radiation dose being 57 times higher than that with CT/SPECT when a four-phases scan is utilized (36). Patient radiation exposure may be lowered with differing protocols; however, these do not achieve rates as low as a sestamibi scan (37).

MULTI-GLAND PARATHYROID DISEASE

Preoperative imaging for the localization of abnormal parathyroid glands is known to be significantly less accurate in patients with MGD due to the relatively smaller gland size when compared to single adenomas (5, 38). In MGD, ultrasound and scintigraphy have been shown to have sensitivity of 35% and 45%, respectively (39). 4D-CT has sensitivity ranging from 45 to 85.7%, with some advocating the use of 4D-CT in patients with higher likelihood of MGD as it most accurately identifies >1 enlarged parathyroid gland (18, 40, 41). Patients known to have or at high risk for MGD should not routinely undergo minimally invasive parathyroidectomy, but should, at minimum, have preoperative thyroid ultrasound to rule out concurrent thyroid pathology (3).

CONCLUSION

In the era of minimally invasive parathyroidectomy, preoperative imaging for the localization of abnormal parathyroid glands is appropriate for patients in whom there is no suspicion of multi-gland parathyroid disease. This includes pediatric patients, although given their age, genetic counseling and testing for a potential familial endocrinopathy, which would influence the timing and extent of parathyroidectomy, are recommended. Prior to planned parathyroidectomy, we routinely obtain both cervical ultrasound and 4D-CT for the preoperative localization of enlarged parathyroid glands and evaluation and work-up of concurrent thyroid nodules, if needed. However, the choice of preoperative imaging study should be determined based on the institutional/local availability of imaging modalities and be guided by institutional data regarding sensitivity, specificity, and expertise in interpreting the obtained studies.

REFERENCES

1. Kollars J, Zarroug AE, van Heerden J, Lteif A, Stavlo P, Suarez L, et al. Primary Hyperparathyroidism in Pediatric Patients. *Pediatrics* 2005;115(4):974–80.
2. Burke JF, Chen H, Gosain A. Parathyroid Conditions in Childhood. *Seminars Pediatric Surg* 2014;23(2):66–70.
3. Wilhelm SM, Wang TS, Ruan DT, Lee JA, Asa SL, Duh Q-Y, et al. The American Association of Endocrine Surgeons Guidelines for Definitive Management of Primary Hyperparathyroidism. *JAMA Surg* 2016;151(10):959–68.
4. Wang TS, Pasieka JL, Carty SE. Techniques of Parathyroid Exploration at North American Endocrine Surgery Fellowship Programs: What the Next Generation is Being Taught. *Am J Surg* 2014;207(4):527–32.
5. Solorzano CC, Carneiro-Pla D. Minimizing cost and Maximizing Success in the Preoperative Localization Strategy for Primary Hyperparathyroidism. *Surg Clinics North Am* 2014;94(3):587–605.
6. Yabuta T, Tsushima Y, Masuoka H, Tomoda C, Fukushima M, Kihara M, et al. Ultrasonographic Features of Intrathyroidal Parathyroid Adenoma Causing Primary Hyperparathyroidism. *Endocr J* 2011;58(11):989–94.
7. Morita SY, Somervell H, Umbricht CB, Dackiw AP, Zeiger MA. Evaluation for Concomitant Thyroid Nodules and Primary Hyperparathyroidism in Patients Undergoing Parathyroidectomy or Thyroidectomy. *Surgery* 2008;144(6):862–6; discussion 6–8.
8. Sidhu S, Campbell P. Thyroid Pathology Associated with Primary Hyperparathyroidism. *Australian NZ J Surg* 2000;70(4):285–7.

9. Wright MC, Jensen K, Mohamed H, Drake C, Mohsin K, Monlezun D, et al. Concomitant Thyroid Disease and Primary Hyperparathyroidism in Patients Undergoing Parathyroidectomy or Thyroidectomy. *Gland Surg* 2017;6(4):368–74.

10. Milas M, Mensah A, Alghoul M, Berber E, Stephen A, Siperstein A, Weber CJ. The Impact of Office Neck Ultrasonography on Reducing Unnecessary Thyroid Surgery in Patients Undergoing Parathyroidectomy. *Thyroid* 2005;15(9):1055–9.

11. Haugen BR, Alexander EK, Bible KC, Doherty GM, Mandel SJ, Nikiforov YE, et al. 2015 American Thyroid Association Management Guidelines for Adult Patients with Thyroid Nodules and Differentiated Thyroid Cancer: The American Thyroid Association Guidelines Task Force on Thyroid Nodules and Differentiated Thyroid Cancer. *Thyroid* 2016;26(1):1–133.

12. Tessler FN, Middleton WD, Grant EG, Hoang JK, Berland LL, Teefey SA, et al. ACR Thyroid Imaging, reporting and Data System (TI-RADS): White Paper of the ACR TI-RADS Committee. *JACR* 2017;14(5):587–95.

13. Haddad RI, Nasr C, Bischoff L, Busaidy NL, Byrd D, Callender G, et al. NCCN Guidelines Insights: Thyroid Carcinoma, Version 2.2018. *J National Compr Cancer Netw* 2018;16(12):1429–40.

14. Gharib H, Papini E, Garber JR, Duick DS, Harrell RM, Hegedus L, et al. American Association of Clinical Endocrinologists, American College of Endocrinology, and Associazione Medici Endocrinologi Medical Guidelines for Clinical Practice for the Diagnosis and Management of Thyroid Nodules--2016 Update. *Endocr Pract* 2016;22(5):622–39.

15. Wang TS, Cheung K, Farrokhyar F, Roman SA, Sosa JA. Would Scan, But Which Scan? A Cost-Utility Analysis to Optimize Preoperative Imaging for Primary Hyperparathyroidism. *Surgery* 2011;150(6):1286–94.

16. Jabiev AA, Lew JI, Solorzano CC. Surgeon-Performed Ultrasound: A Single Institution Experience in Parathyroid Localization. *Surgery* 2009;146(4):569–75; discussion 75–7.

17. Johnson NA, Tublin ME, Ogilvie JB. Parathyroid Imaging: Technique and Role in the Preoperative Evaluation of Primary Hyperparathyroidism. *AJR* 2007;188(6):1706–15.

18. Rodgers SE, Hunter GJ, Hamberg LM, Schellingerhout D, Doherty DB, Ayers GD, et al. Improved Preoperative Planning for Directed Parathyroidectomy with 4-dimensional Computed Tomography. *Surgery* 2006;140(6):932–40; discussion 40–1.

19. Maser C, Donovan P, Santos F, Donabedian R, Rinder C, Scoutt L, Udelsman R. Sonographically Guided Fine Needle Aspiration with Rapid Parathyroid Hormone Assay. *Ann Surg Oncol* 2006;13(12):1690.

20. Norman J, Politz D, Browarsky I. Diagnostic Aspiration of Parathyroid Adenomas Causes Severe Fibrosis Complicating Surgery and final Histologic Diagnosis. *Thyroid* 2007;17(12):1251–5.

21. Agarwal G, Dhingra S, Mishra SK, Krishnani N. Implantation of Parathyroid Carcinoma Along Fine Needle Aspiration Track. *Langenbecks Arch Surg* 2006;391(6):623–6.
22. Alwaheeb S, Rambaldini G, Boerner S, Coiré C, Fiser J, Asa SL. Worrisome Histologic Alterations Following Fine-Needle Aspiration of the Parathyroid. *J Clin Pathol* 2006;59(10):1094–6.
23. Greenspan BS, Dillehay G, Intenzo C, Lavely WC, O'Doherty M, Palestro CJ, et al. SNM Practice Guideline for Parathyroid Scintigraphy 4.0. *J Nucl Med Technol* 2012;40(2):111–8.
24. Chien D, Jacene H. Imaging of Parathyroid Glands. *Otolaryngologic Clinics North Am* 2010;43(2):399–415, x.
25. Eslamy HK, Ziessman HA. Parathyroid Scintigraphy in Patients with Primary Hyperparathyroidism: 99mTc Sestamibi SPECT and SPECT/CT. *RadioGraphics* 2008;28(5):1461–76.
26. Lavely WC, Goetze S, Friedman KP, Leal JP, Zhang Z, Garret-Mayer E, et al. Comparison of SPECT/CT, SPECT, and Planar Imaging with Single- and Dual-Phase (99m)Tc-Sestamibi Parathyroid Scintigraphy. *J Nucl Med* 2007;48(7):1084–9.
27. Slater A, Gleeson FV. Increased Sensitivity and Confidence of SPECT Over Planar Imaging in Dual-Phase Sestamibi for Parathyroid Adenoma Detection. *Clin Nucl Med* 2005;30(1):1–3.
28. Wong KK, Fig LM, Gross MD, Dwamena BA. Parathyroid Adenoma Localization with 99mTc-Sestamibi SPECT/CT: A Meta-Analysis. *Nucl Med Commun* 2015;36(4):363–75.
29. Shafiei B, Hoseinzadeh S, Fotouhi F, Malek H, Azizi F, Jahed A, et al. Preoperative 99mTc-Sestamibi Scintigraphy in Patients with Primary Hyperparathyroidism and Concomitant Nodular Goiter: Comparison of SPECT-CT, SPECT and Planar Imaging. *Eur J Nucl Med Mol Imaging* 2012;39:S371–S.
30. Pata G, Casella C, Besuzio S, Mittempergher F, Salerni B. Clinical Appraisal of 99m Technetium-Sestamibi SPECT/CT Compared to Conventional SPECT in Patients with Primary Hyperparathyroidism and Concomitant Nodular Goiter. *Thyroid* 2010;20(10):1121–7.
31. Hoang JK, Sung W-k, Bahl M, Phillips CD. How to Perform Parathyroid 4D CT: Tips and Traps for Technique and Interpretation. *Radiology* 2014;270(1):15–24.
32. Perrier ND, Edeiken B, Nunez R, Gayed I, Jimenez C, Busaidy N, et al. A Novel Nomenclature to Classify Parathyroid Adenomas. *World J Surg* 2009;33(3):412–6.
33. Kluijfhout WP, Pasternak JD, Beninato T, Drake FT, Gosnell JE, Shen WT, et al. Diagnostic Performance of Computed Tomography for Parathyroid Adenoma Localization; a Systematic Review and Meta-Analysis. *Eur J Radiol* 2017;88:117–28.

34. Hunter GJ, Schellingerhout D, Vu TH, Perrier ND, Hamberg LM. Accuracy of Four-Dimensional CT for the Localization of Abnormal Parathyroid Glands in Patients with Primary Hyperparathyroidism. *Radiology* 2012;264(3):789–95.
35. Yeh R, Tay YD, Tabacco G, Dercle L, Kuo JH, Bandeira L, et al. Diagnostic Performance of 4D CT and Sestamibi SPECT/CT in Localizing Parathyroid Adenomas in Primary Hyperparathyroidism. *Radiology* 2019;291(2):469–76.
36. Mahajan A, Starker LF, Ghita M, Udelsman R, Brink JA, Carling T. Parathyroid Four-Dimensional Computed Tomography: Evaluation of Radiation Dose Exposure During Preoperative Localization of Parathyroid Tumors in Primary Hyperparathyroidism. *World J Surg* 2012;36(6):1335–9.
37. Madorin CA, Owen R, Coakley B, Lowe H, Nam K-H, Weber K, et al. Comparison of Radiation Exposure and Cost Between Dynamic computed Tomography and Sestamibi Scintigraphy for Preoperative Localization of Parathyroid Lesions. *JAMA Surg* 2013;148(6):500–3.
38. Jones JM, Russell CF, Ferguson WR, Laird JD. Pre-operative Sestamibi-Technetium Subtraction Scintigraphy in Primary Hyperparathyroidism: Experience with 156 Consecutive Patients. *Clin Radiol* 2001;56(7):556–9.
39. Ruda JM, Hollenbeak CS, Stack BC, Jr. A systematic Review of the Diagnosis and Treatment of Primary Hyperparathyroidism from 1995 to 2003. *Otolaryngology--Head Neck Surg* 2005;132(3):359–72.
40. Lubitz CC, Hunter GJ, Hamberg LM, Parangi S, Ruan D, Gawande A, et al. Accuracy of 4-Dimensional Computed Tomography in Poorly Localized Patients with Primary Hyperparathyroidism. *Surgery* 2010;148(6):1129–37; discussion 37–8.
41. Starker LF, Mahajan A, Björklund P, Sze G, Udelsman R, Carling T. 4D Parathyroid CT as the Initial Localization Study for Patients with De Novo Primary Hyperparathyroidism. *Ann Surg Oncol* 2011;18(6):1723–8.

11

Hypoparathyroidism in pediatric patients

ANDREW C. CALABRIA AND MICHAEL A. LEVINE

INTRODUCTION

Hypoparathyroidism in children and adolescents may be isolated or part of a complex developmental or autoimmune syndrome. Depending on the severity of the defect in parathyroid development or function, hypoparathyroidism may present in the newborn period, may be transient or permanent, or may not manifest until the child is older. The causes of congenital hypoparathyroidism can be broadly classified into defects that impair formation of the parathyroid glands and those that interfere with normal function of the parathyroid glands; in both cases circulating levels of parathyroid hormone (PTH) will be frankly or inappropriately low in the context of hypocalcemia and hyperphosphatemia. By contrast, biochemical hypoparathyroidism can also be associated with elevated circulating concentration of PTH, particularly in patients with pseudohypoparathyroidism, a condition that is characterized by renal resistance to PTH and which is discussed separately in this edition. Delayed onset of hypoparathyroidism during infancy or childhood might represent an inability of a hypoplastic gland to secrete sufficient PTH to meet the increasing calcium requirements that occur during rapid skeletal growth or during an intercurrent illness. Alternatively, late-onset hypoparathyroidism might reflect accelerated apoptosis of parathyroid cells or development of an autoimmune disorder that leads to destruction of the parathyroid glands. Postsurgical hypoparathyroidism, constituting 75% of all cases in adults, is an unusual cause of hypoparathyroidism in pediatric patients.

ETIOLOGIES

Advances in molecular genetic testing have led to the identification of a growing number of genes that are associated with defects in parathyroid gland development, impaired synthesis or secretion of PTH, and decreased survival of parathyroid glands (see Figure 11.1, Table 11.1, [1]). Genetic defects can be *de novo* or inherited in an autosomal dominant (AD), autosomal recessive (AR), or X-linked recessive pattern.

ISOLATED PARATHYROID APLASIA: *GCM2, SOX3*

Isolated hypoparathyroidism can be caused by genetic defects that impair embryologic development of only the parathyroid glands. The most common form of isolated parathyroid aplasia is due to loss-of-function mutations in the glial cells missing 2 (*GCM2*) gene located at 6p23-24. This gene is considered to be the "master regulator" of parathyroid gland development. In most patients, hypoparathyroidism is due to biallelic mutations that inactivate *GCM2*, and are transmitted in an autosomal recessive manner. On the other hand, some cases show a dominant pattern of inheritance in which *GCM2* mutations produce an abnormal *GCM2* protein with dominant-negative effects. GCM2 is a member of a small family of homologous proteins that regulate gene transcription by interacting with DNA at a unique GCM binding motif. GCM2 is expressed principally if not exclusively in parathyroid cells, and is first detected during early development in the second and third pharyngeal pouches, where it participates as part of a network of transcription factors (e.g., GATA3 and TBX1) that are required for the normal development of the parathyroid gland. Isolated hypoparathyroidism can also be inherited in an X-linked recessive pattern, with affected patients

Genetic Bases for Hypoparathyroidism

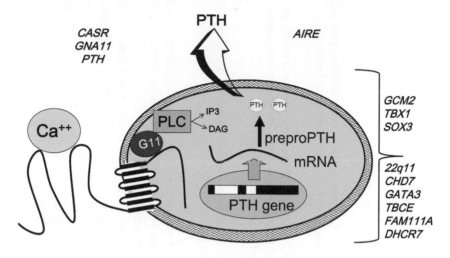

Figure 11.1 Genetic basis for hypoparathyroidism.

presenting with hypocalcemic seizures during infancy. These patients carry mutations at Xq26-27, in which there is a deletion-insertion involving chromosomes 2p25.2 and Xq27.1, near Sry-box 3 (SOX3), which is also thought to impact parathyroid gland development.

COMPLEX DEVELOPMENTAL SYNDROMES ASSOCIATED WITH HYPOPARATHYROIDISM

DiGeorge sequence: 22q11, *TBX1*, 10p13

The DiGeorge sequence (DGS) is a common developmental field defect that includes cardiovascular malformations, hypoparathyroidism, thymic hypoplasia, and characteristic facial and palatal dysmorphism as major clinical features. The triad of congenital absence of the thymus, hypoparathyroidism, and cardiac anomalies, commonly of the outflow tract or aortic arch (i.e., conotruncal defects), was originally described by DiGeorge in 1965. The facial features that have been described in association with 22q11 deletion syndrome include hypertelorism or telecanthus, short or hypoplastic philtrum, cleft palate, micrognathia, and low-set, posteriorly rotated ears. The basic embryological defect is inadequate development of the facial neural crest tissues that result in maldevelopment of third and fourth pharyngeal pouch derivatives. The clinical spectrum of DGS-related disease is highly variable and includes cardiac, thymic, parathyroid, neurologic, behavioral, psychiatric, and craniofacial defects. Various developmental syndromes, with limited features of classic DGS (e.g., velocardiofacial syndrome, Shprintzen syndrome), have also been described as different manifestations of

Table 11.1 Disorders associated with hypoparathyroidism in pediatric patients

Disease	Gene	Locus	OMIM	Associated comorbidities
Disorders of parathyroid gland formation				
Isolated parathyroid aplasia	GCM2	6p23-24	*603716	
	SOX3	Xq-26-27	*307700	
DiGeorge sequence				Thymic hypoplasia with immunodeficiency, cardiac defects, cleft palate, dysmorphic facies
Type 1	TBX1	22q11.21-q11-23	#188400	
Type 2	NEBL	10p13	%601362	
CHARGE syndrome	CHD7	8q12.2	#214800	Cardiac defects, cleft palate, renal anomalies, ear abnormalities/deafness, developmental delay
	SEMA3E	7q21.11	#214800	
Hypoparathyroidism, deafness, renal dysplasia	GATA3	10p14-15	#146255	Deafness and renal dysplasia
Hypoparathyroidism, retardation, dysmorphism (Sanjad–Sakati syndrome)	TBCE	1q42-43	#241410	Growth retardation, developmental delay, dysmorphic facies
Kenny–Caffey syndrome				Short stature, medullary stenosis, dysmorphic facies. Type 1 with developmental delay, whereas Type 2 with normal intelligence
Type 1	TBCE	1q42-43	#244460	
Type 2	FAM111A	11q12.1	#127000	
Smith–Lemli–Opitz syndrome	DHCR7	11q13.4	#270400	Microcephaly, abnormal male genital development, renal dysplasia, syndactyly, adrenal insufficiency, developmental delay

(Continued)

Table 11.1 (Continued) Disorders associated with hypoparathyroidism in pediatric patients

Disease	Gene	Locus	OMIM	Associated comorbidities
Disorders of parathyroid hormone synthesis or secretion				
PTH gene mutations	PTH	11p15.3-p15.1	*168450	
Autosomal dominant hypocalcemia	CASR	3q13.3-q21.1	#601198	Milder phenotype, may not present until second decade
Type 1	GNA11	19p13.3	#615361	Hypercalciuria
Type 2				Short stature; no hypercalciuria
Disorders of parathyroid gland destruction				
Autoimmune polyendocrinopathy candidiasis ectodermal dystrophy	AIRE	21q22.3	#240300	Mucocutaneous candidiasis, adrenal insufficiency, other endocrine diseases (ovarian failure, hypothyroidism, diabetes mellitus, hypophysitis), alopecia, vitiligo, dental enamel hypoplasia

the same molecular defect, typically a large deletion in 22q11. This deletion syndrome is considered the most common human microdeletion, with an incidence of 1 out of 2000 to 4000 births, and is the most common contiguous gene deletion. Hemizygous microdeletions within chromosome 22q11.21-23 are the most common cause of DGS and account for about 85% of cases. Haploinsufficiency of transcription factor *TBX1* has emerged as the likely explanation for the developmental defects of the heart, ears, and parathyroids, but notably not learning disabilities. Small mutations in *TBX1* can cause most of the features of DGS or isolated hypoparathyroidism. A less common basis for DGS is a microdeletion at chromosome 10p.13, called DiGeorge locus type II (DGS2), which includes the likely causal nebulette (*NEBL*) gene, which is expressed in cardiac tissue. DGS can also be caused by fetal exposure to retinoic acid, which inhibits expression of TBX1, or alcohol.

Hypoparathyroidism is present in up to 60% of patients with DGS but is highly variable, and can range from severe, early-onset hypocalcemia with neonatal seizures to mild asymptomatic hypocalcemia that is only discovered later in childhood or even adulthood. Hypoparathyroidism is more common in neonates and infants, especially those with congenital heart disease and receiving concomitant loop diuretics. Hypocalcemia may resolve during childhood, even in some children as young as 1 year of age, but hypoparathyroidism is often latent and can be unmasked during times of stress (e.g., surgery or severe illness), presumably due to insufficient parathyroid reserve (2).

CHARGE syndrome: *CHD7, SEMA3E*

Hypoparathyroidism can be a component of the Coloboma, Heart defects, Atresia choanae, Retarded growth and development, Genital hypoplasia, and Ear anomalies/deafness (CHARGE) syndrome. More than 75% of cases are due to heterozygous loss-of-function mutations in the coding region of the *CHD7* gene at chromosome 8q12.2. *CHD7* is a chromodomain helicase DNA binding protein and is active in chromatin remodeling. Mutations are usually *de novo* but rarely are inherited in an autosomal dominant manner. Less commonly, CHARGE syndrome can be due to abnormalities in semaphoring 3E (Semaphorin 3E), which controls cell positioning during embryonic development on chromosome 7q21.11. There is significant clinical overlap with DGS, as both conditions display hypoparathyroidism, cardiac anomalies, cleft palate, renal anomalies, ear abnormalities/deafness, and developmental delay. In fact, hypoparathyroidism may be more common in newborns with CHARGE syndrome compared to newborns with DGS (3).

Hypoparathyroidism deafness renal dysplasia syndrome: *GATA3*

GATA3, on chromosome 10p14-15, distal to the DGS2 locus, encodes a transcription factor that is expressed not only in the developing parathyroid gland but also thymus, kidney, inner ear, and central nervous system tissues (4). Along with

GCM2 and MafB, two known transcriptional regulators of parathyroid development, GATA3 stimulates the PTH promotor, activating PTH gene transcription and thereby increasing synthesis of PTH. Haploinsufficiency of *GATA3* is associated with hypoparathyroidism, sensorineural deafness, and renal dysplasia (HDR) syndrome, also known as Barakat syndrome, and is inherited in an autosomal dominant pattern. HDR has wide phenotypic variability. Hypoparathyroidism ranges from asymptomatic and transient neonatal hypocalcemia that resolves in infancy to severe symptomatic hypocalcemia with infantile seizures and tetany that requires lifelong treatment. Sensorineural hearing loss, which is often bilateral, is present in more than 95% of HDR patients and is usually identified in infancy or early childhood. Renal dysplasia is present in 60% of patients, but less than 10% of patients have been shown to develop end-stage renal disease. There are no cardiac, immunologic, or palatal abnormalities, which differentiate this syndrome from classical DiGeorge sequence and CHARGE syndrome.

Hypoparathyroidism, retardation, and dysmorphism: *TBCE, FAM111A*

Hypoparathyroidism, retardation, and dysmorphism syndrome, also known as Sanjad–Sakati syndrome, is a rare AR disorder, found almost exclusively in individuals of Arab descent. It is characterized by permanent hypoparathyroidism, severe prenatal and postnatal growth retardation, cognitive impairment, reduced T-cell subsets, and other congenital anomalies, including microcephaly, microphthalmia, micrognathia, ear abnormalities, dental anomalies, and small hands and feet. Kenny–Caffey syndrome (KCS) is a clinically similar allelic syndrome characterized by hypoparathyroidism, severe short stature, thin marrow cavities (medullary stenosis) and thickening of the long bones, and eye abnormalities. Both syndromes map to mutations in the tubulin-specific chaperone E (*TBCE*) gene on chromosome 1q42-43, which encodes a chaperone protein, cofactor E, that with cofactors A, C, and D is involved in the pathway leading to correctly folded β-tubulin from folding intermediates. Cofactor E binds to the cofactor D/β-tubulin complex, and interaction of this complex with cofactor C results in the release of β-tubulin polypeptides that assume proper configuration. Abnormal formation of β-tubulin affects the Golgi apparatus and endosomes, which suggests a possible link between tubulin physiology and parathyroid gland development. KCS can also be inherited in an autosomal dominant fashion, due to a heterozygous mutation of the *FAM111A* gene on chromosome 11q12, which is a chromatin-associated protein involved in DNA replication. Unlike the AR form, individuals with the AD form, termed KCS type 2, have normal intelligence.

Smith–Lemli–Opitz syndrome: *DHCR7*

Hypoparathyroidism due to parathyroid hypoplasia has also been described in some individuals with Smith–Lemli–Opitz syndrome, which is caused by biallelic mutations in the *DHCR7* gene (11q13.4), which encodes delta-7-sterol reductase.

This enzyme catalyzes the final step in cholesterol biosynthesis. Smith–Lemli–Opitz is associated with multiple congenital anomalies, including microcephaly, shortened nose, abnormal male genital development, renal dysplasia, and syndactyly, as well as adrenal insufficiency and mental retardation.

MITOCHONDRIAL DISEASE

Several syndromes that arise from deletions in mitochondrial DNA have also been associated with hypoparathyroidism, but the mechanism(s) by which mitochondrial defects affect parathyroid gland development or function are unknown (5). These primary mitochondrial disorders include the Kearns–Sayre syndrome (encephalomyopathy, ophthalmoplegia, retinitis pigmentosa, heart block), the Pearson marrow-pancreas syndrome (sideroblastic anemia, neutropenia, thrombocytopenia, pancreatic dysfunction), and the maternally inherited diabetes and deafness syndrome. Hypoparathyroidism has also been described in patients with the mitochondrial myopathy, encephalopathy, lactic acidosis, and stroke-like episodes (MELAS) syndrome, owing to point mutations in mitochondrial tRNA. In addition, mutations in the mitochondrial trifunctional protein (MTP) that result in either isolated long-chain 3-hydroxy-acyl-coenzyme A dehydrogenase (LCHAD) deficiency or loss of all three MTP enzymatic activities have been associated with hypoparathyroidism in a few unrelated patients. This condition manifests as hypoketotic hypoglycemia, cardiomyopathy, hepatic dysfunction, and developmental delay and is associated with maternal fatty liver of pregnancy. Medium-chain acyl-CoA dehydrogenase deficiency (MCADD) due to mutations in the *ACADM* gene has also been associated with hypoparathyroidism.

DISORDERS OF PARATHYROID HORMONE SYNTHESIS OR SECRETION

PTH gene mutations

Defects in the *PTH* gene (11p15.3-p15.1) are an uncommon cause of hypoparathyroidism and may arise from AD or AR mutations. Mutations impair the synthesis of preproPTH, 115-amino-acid precursor to mature PTH protein. An autosomal dominant mutation in the signal peptide sequence of preproPTH has been reported to impair the normal processing of preproPTH to PTH, which requires two proteolytic cleavages to occur in order for the biologically active 84-amino-acid mature PTH molecule to be produced and stored in secretory granules. AD mutations disrupt the hydrophobic leader sequence of the nascent peptide, and impair translocation of the abnormal protein across the endoplasmic reticulum (ER). A dominant negative effect is achieved through interference with docking of wild type proteins on the endoplasmic reticulum and/or induction of the ER stress response, which leads to apoptosis of the parathyroid cells. AR forms of PTH gene mutations appear more common, and include splicing defects, missense mutations, and interestingly, defects within the leader sequence of preproPTH.

Autosomal dominant: *CASR, GNA11*

Dominant gain-of-function mutations in the *CASR* gene encoding the calcium-sensing receptor (CASR), or the alpha subunit of the G protein, Gα11 (*GNA11*), that couples CASR to activation of intracellular signaling pathways in the parathyroid cell, result in autosomal dominant hypocalcemia types 1 (ADH1) and 2 (ADH2), respectively (6). In ADH1, heterozygous mutations in the *CASR* increase the sensitivity of the CASR to extracellular ionized calcium, and as a result, PTH synthesis and secretion are inhibited at normal levels of ionized calcium. The presence of the *CASR* mutation in cells of the thick ascending limb of the kidney leads to decreased renal calcium reabsorption, and therefore increased fractional excretion of calcium, with relative or absolute hypercalciuria, is an important biochemical hallmark of this disorder. Most activating mutations of the *CASR* gene on chromosome 3q13.3-q21.1 are familial. In ADH2, increased sensitivity to calcium results from mutations in *GNA11* (19p13) that reduce the threshold for activation of Gα11 by the CASR. Unlike ADH1, ADH2 does not appear to have increased fractional excretion of calcium by the kidney, presumably because Gα11 is not the primary transmembrane coupling protein for the CASR in the distal renal tubule. Individuals with ADH2 have short stature, which is likely due to activated Gα11 signaling in the growth plates of long bones. The clinical presentation of ADH1 and ADH2 is often mild, with many cases not diagnosed until the second decade or later. Nevertheless, some affected patients may manifest clinically symptomatic hypocalcemia, including seizures in the newborn period or infancy. Remarkably, whereas gain-of-function mutations of the *CASR* and *GNA11* genes cause familial hypocalcemia types 1 and 2, respectively, inactivating mutations of the same genes reduce sensitivity of parathyroid cells to extracellular ionized calcium and lead to excessive secretion of PTH and consequent hypercalcemia.

DISORDERS OF PARATHYROID GLAND DESTRUCTION OR INFILTRATION

Autoimmune polyendocrinopathy syndrome type 1: *AIRE*

Hypoparathyroidism can arise due to the development of anti-parathyroid antibodies, so-called "autoimmune hypoparathyroidism." Autoimmune hypoparathyroidism may be isolated or occur in the context of a complex autoimmune syndrome, most commonly the autoimmune polyendocrinopathy candidiasis ectodermal dystrophy (APECED), also known as autoimmune polyglandular syndrome (APS-1). The molecular defect in APS-1 occurs in the autoimmune regulator (*AIRE*) gene at 21q22.3 (7), which encodes a transcription factor that regulates thymic epithelial cells through the transcription of diverse proteins that result in their presentation as self-antigens to developing T cells, with subsequent elimination of autoreactive T cells. Autoantibodies against type 1 interferon are typically present in affected subjects. Most patients have biallelic mutations, but in some patients a non-classical form of APS-1 has been associated with dominant mutations. APECED is an uncommon disorder in most populations (approximately 1:90,000–3:100,000), but it occurs with greater frequency (1:9000 to 1:25,000) in genetically isolated groups such as Finns, Sardinians, and Iranian Jews.

There is wide variability in clinical presentation for affected individuals, without significant genotype–phenoytpe correlation and even significant intrafamilial differences between siblings carrying the same mutation (8). Most cases are detected in early childhood, but some may not present until after the first decade.

The classic triad of APS-1 consists of mucocutaneous candidiasis, hypoparathyroidism, and adrenal insufficiency. The clinical onset of the three principal components of the syndrome typically follows a predictable pattern, in which mucocutaneous candidiasis first appears at a mean age of 5 years, followed by hypoparathyroidism at a mean age of 9 years, and adrenal insufficiency at a mean age of 14 years. Many additional autoimmune features can develop, including endocrinopathies, such as ovarian failure, hypothyroidism, diabetes, and hypophysitis with growth hormone deficiency. Nonendocrine conditions include alopecia, which can start as hairless patches and proceed to alopecia totalis, pernicious anemia, malabsorption, steatorrhea, hepatitis, keratoconjunctivitis, and dystrophic nails. Dental enamel hypoplasia is also common and appears to be unrelated to hypoparathyroidism. Vitiligo, calcifications of the tympanic membranes, and periodic maculopapular, morbilliform, or urticarial rash with fever occur as well as part of the clinical spectrum of APECED. Although most patients with AIRE mutations will manifest multiple features of the APS-1 disorder, some patients with *AIRE* mutations will manifest only hypoparathyroidism.

In APS-1, tissue-specific antibodies directed against the parathyroid, thyroid, and adrenal glands have been identified and support the autoimmune basis. For hypoparathyroidism, antibodies directed against NATCH leucine-rich repeat protein 5 (NALP5) have been identified as the target for autoimmune attack in the parathyroid cells, which leads to tissue destruction. Alternatively, some patients develop antibodies directed against the CASR that activate the receptor and thereby inhibit PTH secretion; hypoparathyroidism may be reversible over time as antibody titers decrease. Autoantibodies against the steroidogenic enzymes (CYP21A2 and CYP17A1) and side chain cleavage enzyme (CYP11A1) are useful markers for the autoimmune destruction of the adrenal cortex even years before the clinical onset of the disease. Autoantibodies to cytochrome CYP11A1 are associated with ovarian insufficiency. T1D is correlated with autoantibodies against insulin, IA-2 tyrosine phosphatase-like protein, and glutamic acid decarboxylase GAD65.

OTHER FORMS OF DESTRUCTIVE HYPOPARATHYROIDISM

Hypoparathyroidism in adults is most commonly seen after surgical excision of or damage to the parathyroid glands after thyroid surgery for thyroid cancer, radical neck dissection for other cancers, typically laryngeal cancer, or repeated operations for primary (or tertiary) hyperparathyroidism. In children, this is a much less common cause of hypoparathyroidism. Transient hypoparathyroidism is seen in up to 30% of all adults, but prolonged hypocalcemia, which may develop immediately or weeks to years after neck surgery, suggests permanent hypoparathyroidism. Rates of hypoparathyroidism after thyroid procedures may be higher in children, but data are limited. A Swedish study reported that 7.3% of patients (n = 274) undergoing total thyroidectomy over a 10-year period had permanent hypoparathyroidism, with longer operative times (>3 hour) noted in affected individuals (9). A single institution study in the United States reported that 37% of patients (n = 137) had transient hypoparathyroidism after total thyroidectomy, but only 2 patients (0.6%) had persistent hypoparathyroidism 6 months after surgery (10). Rarely, hypoparathyroidism occurs in patients who receive extensive radiation to the neck and mediastinum. Hypoparathyroidism is also reported in metal overload diseases such as hemochromatosis and Wilson disease, and in neoplastic or granulomatous infiltration of the parathyroid glands. Hypoparathyroidism may be present in patients with thalassemia who develop iron overload owing to frequent blood transfusion. Hypoparathyroidism has also been observed in association with HIV disease. Children with severe burns can develop hypoparathyroidism, likely due to severe magnesium depletion, with refractoriness to PTH action in target cells and resulting hypocalcemia. Conversely, elevated serum levels of magnesium can directly inhibit PTH secretion via direct interaction with CaSRs.

MANAGEMENT

The management of congenital hypoparathyroidism depends on the presentation of hypocalcemia, which can vary from an asymptomatic biochemical finding to a life-threatening condition. Manifestations of hypocalcemia are due primarily to enhanced neuromuscular excitability (tetany) of the central and peripheral nervous system, and in general reflect the *level* or *rate of decline* of the circulating level of ionized rather than total calcium. Still, in most cases, determination of the total serum calcium level can provide a useful guide to the ionized calcium level, and when plasma protein levels are normal, symptoms and signs of hypocalcemia are common when total calcium concentrations are approximately 7 to 7.5 mg/dL. In addition, the signs and symptoms of hypocalcemic tetany can be amplified by other electrolyte abnormalities, particularly hypomagnesemia and hypokalemia. Patients with chronic hypocalcemia sometimes have few, if any, symptoms of neuromuscular irritability despite markedly decreased serum calcium concentrations. By contrast, patients with acute hypocalcemia frequently manifest many symptoms of tetany. Most patients with hypocalcemia will have some mild features of tetany, including circumoral numbness, paresthesias of the distal extremities, or muscle cramps. Symptoms of fatigue, hyperirritability, anxiety, and depression are also common.

For the acute management of symptomatic hypocalcemia in patients with tetany or cardiovascular manifestations, a slow intravenous injection of 10% calcium gluconate in a dose of 1 to 2 mL/kg up to 10 mL should be started. If tetany persists or recurs, additional intravenous calcium can be administered, preferably as a continuous infusion (1–3 mg/kg/h of elemental calcium). When a continuous infusion of calcium is not feasible, bolus infusions of calcium over several hours, every 6 to 8 hours, may be used, but care must be taken to avoid extravasation of calcium as its precipitation can cause tissue necrosis. Oral therapy with calcium and calcitriol should be instituted as soon as possible to allow discontinuation of intravenous calcium and can help in the transition to daily management of hypoparathyroidism.

Conventional management of chronic hypoparathyroidism includes the use of calcium supplementation and either activated forms of vitamin D or high-dose parent calciferols. Calcium salts should be administered with meals to reduce intestinal absorption of phosphate and reduce serum levels of phosphorus, as well as to provide a consistent daily calcium intake that will minimize fluctuations in serum calcium that might arise from day-to-day differences in dietary calcium intake. The administration of calcium with meals also avoids the problem of reduced enteral absorption that occurs when gastric acid secretion is reduced. Oral calcium supplements come in liquid or tablet preparations and are most commonly available as calcium carbonate and calcium citrate. Calcium carbonate contains 40% elemental calcium by weight, and therefore fewer and smaller tablets are required. Some patients will develop constipation from calcium carbonate, and for those individuals alternatives such as calcium citrate (20% elemental calcium) can be considered. The goal of long-term treatment is to maintain the plasma calcium concentration in the slightly low to low normal range, about 8.0 to 9.0 mg/dL, and a calcium × phosphorus product of less than 55 mg^2/dL^2 to avoid hypercalciuria. The plasma phosphorus concentration also decreases as the serum calcium level is raised, but this decrease lags behind the rise of plasma calcium and often some degree of hyperphosphatemia may persist. Presumably because of the normal or elevated levels of serum phosphorus that maintain an elevated calcium × phosphorus product, mineralization defects do not occur in hypoparathyroidism, as in rickets, where hypophosphatemia is felt to be the basis for growth plate defects.

In addition to calcium supplementation, conventional treatment will require the administration of vitamin D. Vitamin D analogs that possess a 1-α-hydroxyl group, such as natural 1,25(OH)2D3 (calcitriol) or the 1 alpha-hydroxylated analog, 1alpha(OH)D3 (which after 25-hydroxylation in the liver is converted to 1,25[OH]2D3), do not require activation by PTH, and thus are most suitable for the treatment of hypoparathyroidism. Chronic treatment with calcitriol will usually require doses of 0.025 to 0.05 mcg/kg/day in two divided doses, but much greater doses may be necessary when therapy is first initiated. Children with hypoparathyroidism are at significant risk for treatment-related hypercalciuria and nephrocalcinosis. Plasma and urinary calcium, as well as serum phosphorus, should be regularly monitored to achieve a steady state in which patients are essentially free of symptoms and signs of hypocalcemia and do not have hypercalciuria. Renal ultrasound should be performed every 1 to 2 years to identify kidney stones or nephrocalcinosis.

Studies of PTH replacement in both adults and children with hypoparathyroidism show promise but also reveal limitations. Specifically, data are limited in children, and given the theoretical increased risk for osteosarcoma in individuals with open growth plates, recombinant forms of PTH are only approved in adults. PTH(1-34), given by two or three subcutaneous injections per day or by continuous subcutaneous infusion, has been used safely, with normal or slightly below normal serum calcium levels, for up to 10 years in children with different forms of hypoparathyroidism (e.g., APS-1, CASR) (11). However, this, and other studies, have shown differential effects on skeletal compartments; nearly half had progression of baseline nephrocalcinosis, and after discontinuation, many exhibited increased calcium and calcitriol requirements, suggestive of hungry bone syndrome. The clinical use of PTH(1-84) remains limited in children but is approved for adults with hypoparathyroidism who cannot be well controlled on conventional therapy with calcium and calcitriol. This is based in part on a double-blind, randomized controlled study of adults (n = 134) receiving PTH(1-84) in which just over half subjects achieved a 50% reduction of calcium and calcitriol requirements while maintaining goal calcium levels (12).

SUMMARY

Hypoparathyroidism in children can present in isolation or as part of a developmental syndrome. Technological advances in molecular testing have increasingly recognized genetic causes of hypoparathyroidism and have helped to elucidate mechanisms for parathyroid gland development, synthesis and secretion of PTH, and destruction of the parathyroid glands. The increased availability of commercially available genetic panels has allowed for more cost-effective and efficient testing for putative genes. Accurate diagnosis of the underlying genetic diagnosis remains essential, and this allows for screening for potential comorbidities, establishment of treatment goals, and for additional family planning.

REFERENCES

1. Gordon RJ, Levine MA. Genetic Disorders of Parathyroid Development and Function. *Endocrinol Metab Clin N Am* 2018;47(4):809–23.
2. Fujii S, Nakanishi T. Clinical Manifestations and Frequency of Hypocalcemia in 22q11.2 Deletion Syndrome. *Pediat Int* 2015;57(6):1086–9.
3. Jyonouchi S, McDonald-McGinn DM, Bale S, Zackai EH, Sullivan KE. CHARGE (Coloboma, Heart Defect, Atresia Choanae, Retarded Growth and Development, Genital Hypoplasia, Ear Anomalies/Deafness) Syndrome and Chromosome 22q11.2 Deletion Syndrome: A Comparison of Immunologic and Nonimmunologic Phenotypic Features. *Pediatrics* 2009;123(5):e871–7.

4. Van Esch H, Groenen P, Nesbit MA, et al. GATA3 Haplo-Insufficiency Causes Human HDR Syndrome. *Nature* 2000;406(6794):419–22.
5. Chow J, Rahman J, Achermann JC, Dattani MT, Rahman S. Mitochondrial Disease and Endocrine Dysfunction. *Nat Rev Endocrinol* 2017;13(2):92–104.
6. Roszko KL, Bi RD, Mannstadt M. Autosomal Dominant Hypocalcemia (Hypoparathyroidism) Types 1 and 2. *Front Physiol* 2016;7:458.
7. DeMartino L, Capalbo D, Improda N, et al. Novel Findings into AIRE Genetics and Functioning: Clinical implications. *Front Pediatr* 2016;4(86):1–8.
8. Capalbo D, Mazza C, Giordano R, et al. Molecular Background and Genotype-Phenotype Correlation in Autoimmune-Polyendocrinopathy-Candidiasis-Ectodermal Dystrophy Patients from Campania and in Their Relatives. *J Endocrinol Invest* 2012;35(2):169–73.
9. Nordenstrom E, Bergenfelz A, Almquist M. Permanent Hypoparathyroidism After Total Thyroidectomy in Children: Results from a National Registry. *World J Surg* 2018;42(9):2858–63.
10. Baumgarten HD, Bauer AJ, Isaza A, et al. Surgical Management of Pediatric Thyroid Disease: Complication Rates After Thyroidectomy at the Children's Hospital of Philadelphia High-Volume Pediatric Thyroid Center. *J Pediatr Surg* 2019;54(10):1969–75.
11. Winer KK, Kelly A, Johns A, Zhang B, Dowdy K, Kim L, et al. Long-Term Parathyroid Hormone 1–34 Replacement Therapy in Children with Hypoparathyroidism. *J Pediatr* 2018;203:391–9.
12. Rubin MR, Cusano NE, Fan WW, Delgado Y, Zhang C, Costa AG, et al. Therapy of Hypoparathyroidism With PTH(1–84): A Prospective Six Year Investigation of Efficacy and Safety. *J Clin Endocrinol Metab* 2016;101(7):2742–50.

12

Pseudohypoparathyroidism

AMBIKA P. ASHRAF AND TODD D. NEBESIO

INTRODUCTION

Pseudohypoparathyroidism (PHP) and related disorders represent a form of hormone resistance related to abnormalities in the activation of G proteins. G proteins are a superfamily of heterotrimeric guanine nucleotide binding proteins composed of three functionally distinct subunits (α, β, γ). The hormones that activate the G protein include glycoproteins (TSH, FSH, and LH), peptides (PTH, PTHrP, ACTH, CRH, GHRH, glucagon, GLP, GIP), and neurotransmitters (norepinephrine, melanocortin, and dopamine).

The interaction between these hormones and their specific G protein coupled receptors activates the α-subunit of the stimulatory G protein (Gsα, encoded by *GNAS*) leading to dissociation of the α-subunit of the heterotrimeric stimulatory G protein from the β and γ subunits. The activation by Gsα of adenylyl cyclase leads to synthesis of the intracellular messenger cyclic AMP (cAMP). Protein kinase A (PKA) is a primary target of cAMP, and the binding of cAMP to Type 1 Regulatory Subunit 1 Alpha (PRKAR1A) results in a cascade of intracellular events, including the phosphorylation of phosphodiesterases (PDEs), such as PDE4D. Figure 12.1 illustrates the cAMP-mediated signaling pathway. The underlying molecular defect in PHP varies from lack of activation at the receptor through molecular defects affecting the Gsα or abnormalities in the downstream signaling pathways, namely PRKAR1A and PDE4D (Gsα/cAMP/PKA pathway) (1).

This related heterogeneous group of disorders varies in the severity of the end organ resistance to multiple G protein hormones that activate cAMP through Gsα, primarily PTH, but also may include TSH, gonadotropins (LH/FSH), and GHRH. Collectively, this group is commonly termed "inactivating PTH/PTHrP signaling disorder" (iPPSD) (2).

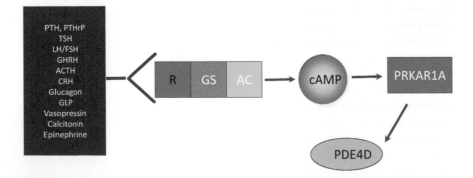

Figure 12.1 The activated Gsα interacts with adenylyl cyclase, promoting the production of cAMP, which interacts with the regulatory subunit and activates downstream signaling pathways, namely PRKAR1A and PDE4D. Abbreviations: R—receptor, GS—G protein stimulatory unit, AC—adenyl cyclase, PRKAR1A—protein kinase type 1α regulatory subunit, PDE4D—phosphodiesterase.

MOLECULAR GENETICS

GNAS, the gene that encode Gsα, is an imprinted gene that maps to chromosome 20q13 and contains 13 exons (3). In most tissues, there is biallelic expression of maternal and paternal Gsα alleles that are encoded by the *GNAS* exons. However, in some specific human tissues (e.g., proximal renal tubules, pituitary gland, gonads, and thyroid), there is tissue-specific imprinting, with the Gsα preferentially expressed from the maternal allele (4). This tissue-specific monoallelic expression of Gsα explains most of the clinical outcomes that depend on the parental origin of the *GNAS* mutation.

Categories of PHP and related disorders:

1. PHP type 1A (PHP1A): heterozygous inactivating mutation in the *GNAS* gene encoding for Gsα is the most common cause of PHP. Loss of maternal imprinting (lack of expression of maternal allele) leads to defective function of Gsα in the target tissues that has maternal tissue-specific imprinting (e.g., proximal renal tubules [PTH], pituitary gland [GHRH], gonads [LH/FSH], and thyroid [TSH]). Features of Albright hereditary osteodystrophy (AHO) are common in PHP1A.
2. PHP type 1B (PHP1B): abnormal patterns of methylation (loss of imprinting) in the differentially methylated regions (DMR) associated with *GNAS* complex locus at the maternal exon (*GNAS A/B*: TSS-DMR). There is also a paternal-specific imprinting pattern of *GNAS* DMR on both alleles resulting in a clinical phenotype characterized by renal resistance to PTH and mild resistance to TSH in the absence of other endocrine or physical abnormalities (no AHO features) and normal Gsα activity.
3. PHP type 1C (PHP1C): lack of expression of maternal allele and characterized by multi-hormone resistance and the presence of signs of AHO. Normal Gsα activity. Considered a variant of PHP type 1A.
4. Pseudopseudohypoparathyroidism (PPHP): paternally derived inactivating mutations in *GNAS* gene (lack of expression of paternal allele). AHO phenotype occurs in the absence of endocrine abnormalities.
5. Progressive osseous heteroplasia (POH): paternally inherited *GNAS* inactivating mutations. Characterized by ectopic bone formation in dermis, skeletal muscle, and deep connective tissues. No PTH resistance.
6. Genetic alterations within *PRKAR1A* and *PDE4D*: heterozygous point mutations in either gene cause acrodysostosis (brachydactyly involving all phalanxes, metacarpals, and metatarsals), nasal hypoplasia, facial dysostosis, and variable hormone resistance (e.g., PTH and TSH).
7. PHP type 2 (PHP2): molecular defect has not been identified.

GNAS genetic defects are most commonly inherited in an autosomal dominant mode. Spontaneous mutations can also occur. There is a significant molecular overlap between these disorders with classical mutations at the GNAS complex gene, complex epigenetic alterations, and mutations in the *PRKAR1A* and *PDE4D* genes (5).

PHP1A occurs only in children of an obligate female carrier (i.e., mother with PHP1A or PPHP), whereas men with either condition have children affected by only PPHP. Affected patients have a 50% chance of transmitting the molecular defect, and depending on their sex, the descendant will develop PPHP or POH (when the patient is male) or PHP1A or PHP1C (when the patient is female).

CLINICAL FINDINGS

Patients with PHP can have a wide spectrum of clinical manifestations that vary in presentation and severity (Table 12.1).

FEATURES OF AHO

Physical features of AHO are most commonly associated with PHP1A, PHP1C, and PPHP. The clinical findings of AHO include a *round face, short stature, heterotopic ossifications, brachydactyly, early-onset obesity, and variable degrees of intellectual disability and developmental delays.*

Short stature: most patients with PHP are short as children and short as adults. However, height in early childhood can be normal. As these children age, there is a decline in growth velocity and diminished pubertal growth spurt (6). Many patients with PHP1A develop GHRH resistance and GH deficiency. Skeletal maturation is frequently advanced, and there is early epiphyseal closure (Figure 12.2), which accounts for part of the short stature independent of GHRH resistance.

Heterotopic ossifications: patients can present with calcified nodules in the dermis and subcutaneous tissue due to a developmental defect resulting from Gsα deficiency in mesenchymal stem cells. These lesions occur most commonly in POH and PPHP, but they can occur to variable degrees in PHP1A and PHP1B. Ectopic ossification is unrelated to serum levels of calcium or phosphorus. Ectopic ossifications are a specific sign of *GNAS* mutations, particularly when observed at birth or in early childhood.

Brachydactyly (Figure 12.2): shortening of III, IV, V metacarpals (brachymetacarpia) and I distal phalanx (bracytelephalangy). This is due to premature closure of the growth plate due to impaired PTHrP signaling in chondrocytes resulting from Gsα deficiency. It is usually absent at birth, but it typically becomes apparent during childhood and more noticeable before puberty.

Early onset obesity is frequently observed. Compared to controls, affected children have decreased resting energy expenditure as well as hyperphagic symptoms. As they get older, these features become less pronounced, and obesity is less severe in adulthood. Sleep disturbances, including sleep apnea, are increased in individuals with PHP.

Intellectual disabilities and developmental delays are common but can vary amongst patients. About 80% of patients with PHP1A have cognitive impairment but only 10% of those with PPHP have problems (7).

Table 12.1 Classification and characteristics of the various types of pseudohypoparathyroidism

PHP	Type 1a	Type 1b	Type 1c	PPHP	Type 2
Molecular abnormality	Mutation in the coding sequence of GNAS (maternal allele)	Abnormal methylation of GNAS A/B:TSS-DMR Deletion at STX16 gene	Mutation in the coding sequence of GNAS (maternal allele) (exon 13 preferentially)	Mutation in the coding sequence of GNAS (paternal allele)	
Gsα mutations	Maternal inheritance	Isolated imprinting dysregulation	None	Paternal inheritance	None
Hormone resistance	PTH, TSH, GHRH, prolactin, gonadotropins Calcitonin	PTH, TSH, calcitonin	PTH, TSH, gonadotropins, glucagon	None	None
AHO phenotype	Yes	No	Yes	Yes	No
Administration of PTH	No renal cAMP production No phosphaturic response	No renal cAMP production No phosphaturic response	Normal urine cAMP No phosphaturic response	Normal renal cAMP production Normal phosphaturic response	Normal renal cAMP production No phosphaturic response

Legend: PHP: pseudohypoparathyroidism; PPHP: pseudopseudohypoparathyroidism; AHO: Albright hereditary osteodystrophy.

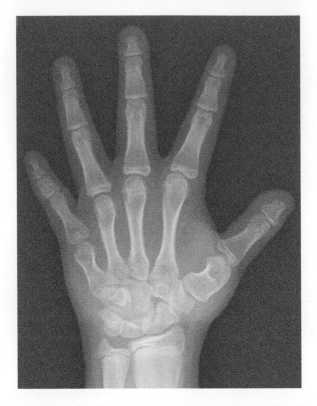

Figure 12.2 Bone age of a 12-year-old male with PHP1A. Skeletal age is 16 years or 4 years advanced. All of the growth plates in the metacarpals are fused. Many of the metacarpal bones are shortened and thickened.

CLINICAL EVALUATION OF PATIENTS WITH PHP

- Short stature (height, growth velocity). Linear growth may initially be normal, but eventual short stature is common.
- Obesity (weight, BMI).
- Dysmorphic facial features.
- Brachydactyly.
- Abnormal dentition.
- Subcutaneous ossifications.
- Developmental and psychoeducational evaluation.
- Lack of pubertal development or diminished pubertal growth spurt.
- Findings consistent with acute or chronic hypocalcemia include paresthesia, muscle cramps, tetany, hyperreflexia, or seizures. Hypocalcemia can clinically be detected as a positive Chvostek sign (twitching of facial muscles after tapping the facial nerve just in front of the ear) and/or Trousseau sign (carpal spasm after maintaining an arm blood pressure cuff at 20 mm Hg above the patient's systolic blood pressure for 3 minutes).

- Ectopic calcification. Patients may develop ectopic calcification in areas such as the gray-white cerebral intersection of brain and basal ganglia, as well as cataracts due to elevated calcium-phosphate product.

BIOCHEMICAL FINDINGS

PTH resistance

PTH resistance is absent at birth, but it gradually develops during infancy or childhood. A high serum phosphorous and elevated PTH are the first biochemical features, and later followed by serum calcium reduction. However, it may take up to 5 years or more before the onset of hypocalcemia (8). Patients develop hyperphosphatemia, low 1,25-dihydroxyvitamin D (1,25[OH]$_2$D), and reduced serum calcium.

In the renal proximal tubule, PTH resistance leads to reduced generation of active 1,25(OH)$_2$D by the loss of the transcriptional induction of 1-alpha hydroxylase, which in turn leads to reduced expression of sodium-dependent phosphate transporters in the renal tubule, lack of phosphaturia, and development of hyperphosphatemia. In the distal tubule, affected patients have appropriate CaSR function and thus can reabsorb calcium appropriately. In the intestine, calcium absorption is reduced due to the defect in the generation of 1,25(OH)$_2$D.

PHP2 is characterized by an increase in levels of cAMP in response to exogenous PTH infusion but a deficient phosphaturic response. Even though the molecular defect has not been identified, PHP2 is associated with vitamin D deficiency. Other possibilities to explain PHP2 are defective signaling downstream of Gsα (9).

RESISTANCE TO OTHER HORMONES

TSH resistance occasionally manifests as elevated TSH levels in the neonatal period, but it more often develops later in childhood or adolescence. Patients can have mild to moderately elevated TSH levels, normal to slightly low free thyroxine levels, no goiter, and negative thyroid autoantibodies. In a newborn with congenital hypothyroidism but a normal thyroid gland, the diagnosis of PHP should be considered if phenotypic features are present.

Gonadotropin resistance can manifest as delayed or incomplete sexual maturation, menstrual irregularities, or infertility in females. Males can present with cryptorchidism and/or lack of a pubertal growth spurt.

GHRH resistance can present as deficient GH secretion and short stature.

Additional hormonal defects described in small series of PHP patients include prolactin deficiency, blunted plasma cAMP responses to glucagon and isoproterenol, resistance to calcitonin, and reduced insulin sensitivity.

Patients with acrodysostosis due to mutations in *PRKAR1A* have universal resistance to PTH, and nearly all have TSH resistance. Only a small subset of individuals with acrodysostosis due to mutations in *PDE4D* have PTH and/or TSH resistance. There is a significant overlap between different but related disorders affecting the cAMP pathway.

LABORATORY/RADIOGRAPHIC EVALUATION OF PATIENTS WITH PSEUDOHYPOPARATHYROIDISM

- PTH resistance: low calcium, elevated PTH, and elevated phosphorus. Serum concentrations of 25(OH)D and 1,25(OH)D2 should also be checked.
- TSH resistance: elevated TSH with normal to low free thyroxine.
- GHRH resistance: low IGF-1 levels are suggestive of GH deficiency. Provocative GH stimulation testing may be abnormal and consistent with GH deficiency.
- Gonadotropin resistance: baseline gonadotropin levels usually are not helpful as they can be normal in patients with menstrual irregularities and hypogonadism.
- Bone age is often significantly advanced along with shortened metacarpals.
- Bone density is usually increased. Due to the selective involvement of PTH in the proximal renal tubule, patients with PHP1B without skeletal resistance to PTH at the bone can develop parathyroid bone disease. Long-standing secondary hyperparathyroidism with chronic hypocalcemia and $1,25(OH)_2D$ deficiency has been associated with tertiary hyperparathyroidism in these patients.

DIAGNOSIS

PHP is often diagnosed clinically and with laboratory tests. Table 12.2 details the diagnostic criteria for PHP. The diagnosis can be confirmed by molecular genetic analysis.

- Sequence analysis of exons 1 through 13 of *GNAS* locus should be performed first, followed by gene-targeted deletion/duplication analysis if no pathogenic variant is found (4).
- Patients with PTH resistance and/or features of AHO, in the absence of subcutaneous ossifications, may be evaluated by targeted sequence analysis of different genes, e.g., *GNAS*, *PRKAR1A*, *PTHLH*, *PDE4D*, and *PDE3A*.
- Methylation analysis at the *GNAS A/B*:TSS-DMR can be performed in patients who present with PTH resistance without features of AHO (PHP1B/iPPSD3, i.e., an imprinting defect) or in patients with PHP1A who do not have a mutation in those *GNAS* exons encoding Gsα.
- In familial PHP1B, evaluate for *STX16* deletion.
- Patients with PHP for whom no molecular cause has been identified (<10%) through these diagnostic approaches may benefit from exome and/or whole-genome sequencing.

Table 12.2 Diagnostic criteria for PHP

1. Clinical features

Features of AHO

a) **Major criteria**: brachydactyly, and short stature, reduced growth velocity (in children).

b) **Additional criteria**: round face, stocky build, obesity, ectopic ossifications (either clinically evident or on radiology studies).

2. Biochemical features

a) **Major laboratory findings**: PTH resistance: raised serum PTH levels with hypocalcemia and hyperphosphatemia in the absence of vitamin D deficiency, magnesium deficiency, and normal renal function.

b) **Additional laboratory findings**: TSH resistance: raised serum TSH levels, usually in the absence of anti-thyroid antibodies.

Resistance to gonadotropins: variable, baseline gonadotropin and sex steroid levels are often normal.

GHRH resistance: blunted GH response to provocative tests.

MANAGEMENT

Patients should be screened at diagnosis and during follow-up for specific features related to hormone resistance (9).

MANAGEMENT OF PTH RESISTANCE

The objective in the management of PTH resistance is to maintain calcium and phosphorus levels in the normal range, which is different than typical hypoparathyroidism where calcium levels are targeted to lower levels. The goal PTH level is to be in the upper part or slightly above the reference range. There is concern that elevated PTH levels may cause bone and mineralization problems, but many affected patients have PTH resistance at the level of the bone. In PHP1B, it is important to normalize PTH in order to prevent irreversible hyperparathyroidism and to reduce bone resorption. Avoidance of PTH suppression is also important, as this can result in hypercalciuria and nephrocalcinosis.

- Regular monitoring of serum levels of calcium, phosphorus, and PTH every 6 months in children and at least yearly in adults.
- Serum levels of 25(OH) vitamin D should be maintained within the normal range.
- Current guidelines recommend checking urinary calcium and renal imaging studies. However, as there is normal activity at the distal convoluted tubule in the kidney to reabsorb calcium, the risks of hypercalciuria and nephrocalcinosis in those with normal serum calcium levels are low (10).

- Treatment involves activated vitamin D (calcitriol or 1,25[OH]$_2$D).
- Calcium carbonate is used to bind and lower serum phosphorus levels.
- Dietary intake of phosphorus (dairy products and meats) in individuals with persistently elevated serum phosphate levels should be limited.
- Adequate management of PTH resistance to reduce the calcium-phosphate product to less than 55 may reduce the development or worsening of calcifications in the lens and brain. However, treatment has no effect on heterotopic ossification.

MANAGEMENT OF TSH RESISTANCE

Treatment of hypothyroidism is by levothyroxine administration to achieve a normal TSH level.

MANAGEMENT OF SHORT STATURE

- Patients with PHP and short stature or decreased growth velocity may have GH deficiency. Early provocative GH testing is important for PHP1A and PPHP patients since epiphyses can fuse prematurely (11). Treatment with GH is effective in improving linear growth in prepubertal children with PHP (12).
- Some children with PHP are born small for gestational age (SGA), specifically in PPHP and forms of acrodysostosis, and they may qualify for GH under the FDA-approved indication for SGA.
- Bone age is usually significantly advanced, which may ultimately lead to reduced final adult height.

MANAGEMENT OF GONADOTROPIN RESISTANCE

Hypogonadism in males and females is treated with testosterone and estrogen/progesterone, respectively.

PREVENTION OF OBESITY

Dietary and lifestyle measures should be implemented at the time of diagnosis, irrespective of the body mass index. Patients should be screened at diagnosis and during follow-up for weight gain, glucose intolerance or type 2 diabetes mellitus, and hypertension.

HETEROTOPIC OSSIFICATIONS

There is currently no specific therapy or medication for heterotopic ossifications. Small ossifications usually do not progress. Ossifications that cause pain and/or irritations may be surgically removed. Regular limb mobilization and physical therapy are necessary when ossifications surround joints.

OPHTHALMOLOGIC EVALUATION

Monitoring for cataracts is important, especially when calcium and phosphorus levels are elevated.

NEUROCOGNITIVE IMPAIRMENT

Developmental delays, intellectual, and learning disabilities are common. Performance IQ is usually more affected than verbal IQ. School assistance and educational support are often required. Developmental therapies (e.g., physical, occupational, and speech therapy) can be beneficial.

DENTAL EVALUATION

Failure of tooth eruption, short blunted roots, dental pulp alterations, hypodontia, and enamel hypoplasia can occur. Regular dental examinations every 6 to 12 months during childhood are recommended.

It is important to consider evaluation in apparently asymptomatic first-degree relatives of an affected individual in order to identify as early as possible those who would benefit from prompt initiation of treatment.

REFERENCES

1. Mantovani G, Elli FM. Multiple Hormone Resistance and Alterations of G-Protein-Coupled Receptors Signaling. *Best Pract Res Clin Endocrinol Metab* 2018 Apr;32(2):141–54.
2. Turan S. Current Nomenclature of Pseudohypoparathyroidism: Inactivating Parathyroid Hormone/Parathyroid Hormone-Related Protein Signaling Disorder. *J Clin Res Pediatr Endocrinol* 2017;9(Suppl 2):58.
3. Gejman PV, Weinstein LS, Martinez M, Spiegel AM, Cao Q, Hsieh WT, et al. Genetic Mapping of the Gs-alpha Subunit Gene (GNAS1) to the Distal Long Arm of Chromosome 20 Using a Polymorphism Detected by Denaturing Gradient Gel Electrophoresis. *Genomics* 1991 Apr;9(4):782–3.
4. Haldeman-Englert CR, Hurst AC, Levine MA. Disorders of GNAS inactivation. *GeneReviews* 1993. Available at: https://www.ncbi.nlm.nih.gov/books/NBK459117/.
5. Linglart A, Levine MA, Juppner H. Pseudohypoparathyroidism. *Endocrinol Metab Clin North Am* 2018 Dec;47(4):865–88.
6. De Wijn E, Steendijk R. Growth and Maturation in Pseudo-Hypoparathyroidism; a Longitudinal Study in 5 Patients. *Eur J Endocrinol* 1982;101(2):223–6.
7. Mouallem M, Shaharabany M, Weintrob N, Shalitin S, Nagelberg N, Shapira H, et al. Cognitive Impairment is Prevalent in Pseudohypoparathyroidism Type Ia, but Not in pseudopseudohypoparathyroidism: Possible Cerebral Imprinting of Gsα. *Clin Endocrinol* 2008;68(2):233–9.

8. Gelfand IM, Eugster EA, DiMeglio LA. Presentation and Clinical Progression of Pseudohypoparathyroidism With Multi-Hormone Resistance and Albright Hereditary Osteodystrophy: A Case Series. *J Pediatr* 2006;149(6):877–80. e1.

9. Mantovani G, Bastepe M, Monk D, De Sanctis L, Thiele S, Usardi A, et al. Diagnosis and Management of Pseudohypoparathyroidism and Related Disorders: First International Consensus Statement. *Nat Rev Endocrinol* 2018;14(8):476.

10. Hansen DW, Nebesio TD, DiMeglio LA, Eugster EA, Imel EA. Prevalence of Nephrocalcinosis in Pseudohypoparathyroidism: Is Screening Necessary? *J Pediatr* 2018;199:263–6.

11. Germain-Lee EL. Management of Pseudohypoparathyroidism. *Curr Opin Pediatr* 2019 Aug;31(4):537–49.

12. Mantovani G, Ferrante E, Giavoli C, Linglart A, Cappa M, Cisternino M, et al. Recombinant Human GH Replacement Therapy in Children with Pseudohypoparathyroidism Type Ia: First Study on the Effect on Growth. *J Clin Endocrinol Metab* 2010;95(11):5011–7.

13

Other genetic parathyroid conditions

TAL YALON AND HAGGI MAZEH

INTRODUCTION

Hyperparathyroidism (HPT) is an uncommon cause of hypercalcemia in the pediatric population. Primary hyperparathyroidism (PHPT) is an endocrine disorder characterized by an autonomous pathological secretion of parathyroid hormone (PTH) by one or more parathyroid glands leading to hypercalcemia. Although common in adults with an estimated prevalence of up to 0.86%, it is a rare cause of hypercalcemia in the pediatric population with reported incidence of 2–5 per 100,000, and accounts for 1% of hypercalcemia cases (1, 2).

In most cases PHPT is sporadic, with no familial history of HPT or relation to other endocrinopathies. It is estimated that in the general population, about 10% of cases of PHPT are a result of hereditary cases and associated with germline mutation in 1 of 11 genes. The suspicion of a genetic cause for PHPT rises even higher in young patients, especially with a familial history of hypercalcemia (3). From a practical stand point, it is recommended by the American Association of Endocrine Surgeons (AAES) Guidelines for Definitive Management of PHPT that genetic counseling should be performed for patients younger than 40 years with PHPT and multi-gland disease (MGD) and considered for those with a family history or syndromic manifestations (4).

Familial PHPT are a group of inherited disorders, mostly in an autosomal dominant manner, and can be isolated or related to other endocrinopathies. In general, they can be divided into syndromic and non-syndromic causes. In this chapter we will elaborate on these entities.

SYNDROMIC CAUSES OF PRIMARY HYPERPARATHYROIDISM

Multiple endocrine neoplasia (MEN) syndromes

Multiple endocrine neoplasia (MEN) are a group of autosomal dominant inherited disorders in which patients have a tendency to develop two or more endocrine tumors, each with distinctive features. PHPT can manifest in patients with MEN-1, MEN-2A, and MEN-4.

Multiple endocrine neoplasia (MEN) 1

MEN-1 is an autosomal dominant inherited (and rarely sporadic) syndrome with a high degree of penetrance that predisposes to tumors of the parathyroid gland, anterior pituitary gland, and entero-pancreatic endocrine cells (also remembered by the 3Ps: parathyroid, pituitary, and pancreas). These develop in 90%, 30–70%, and 30–40% of patients, respectively, by age 40. In addition these patient are at risk for thymic and bronchial neuroendocrine tumors, gastric enterochromaffin-like tumors, and adrenal tumors (5). First described by Dr. Paul Wermer in 1953, it is estimated to have a prevalence of 2–3/100,000. The *MEN1* gene, discovered in 1997, is a tumor suppressor gene, located on the long arm of chromosome 11 (11q13), and codes for the 610 amino acid nuclear protein called Menin. With more than 1000 identified somatic and germline mutations, the exact mechanism by which mutation to this protein causes endocrine tumors remains unknown (6).

MEN-1 is the most common familial form of PHPT. Some of the unique clinical features of PHPT in MEN-1 patients are earlier age of onset (age 20–25 years compared with above 50 years in sporadic cases), equal gender distribution, and higher likelihood of developing multiglandular disease throughout life. It is recommended that these patients be screened annually, from the age of 8 years, for PHPT by a biochemical profile that includes serum calcium and PTH measurements. Once the diagnosis of PHPT is established, it is recommended to advance towered surgical treatment. Since there is a high rate of recurrence due to a development of multiglandular disease, even if not found on initial presentation, it is recommended to perform bilateral parathyroid exploration with subtotal parathyroidectomy (i.e., removal of 3–3.5 glands) or a total parathyroidectomy with immediate auto-transplantation (4, 7).

MULTIPLE ENDOCRINE NEOPLASIA (MEN) 2A

Classical MEN-2A is a familial syndrome characterized by medullary thyroid cancer (MTC), pheochromocytoma, and parathyroid tumors with a penetrance of 99%, 50%, and 20–30%, respectively. First described by Dr. John H. Sipple in 1961, it is an inherited autosomal dominant trait of a mutation of the *RET* gene. The *RET* protooncogene, discovered in 1988, is localized on chromosome 10 (10q11.2) and encodes a transmembrane tyrosine kinase receptor expressed by cells of neural crest origin: the C cells of the thyroid, adrenal medullary cells, and enteric autonomic ganglion cells (3, 8). It is found in 95% of patients with MEN-2A with a strong genotype–phenotype correlation classified into four risk levels for a prophylactic thyroidectomy for the prevention of MTC.

The usual onset of PHPT in MEN-2A patients occurs at the mean age of 38 years, with 5% of patients experiencing hypercalcemic manifestation before any other presentation. The course is usually indolent and rarely requires treatment in childhood (6, 8). Typically, there is an asymmetric hyperplasia of the parathyroid glands, and the surgical treatment strategy recommended by the AAES guidelines is resection of only visibly enlarged glands. If all glands are abnormal, subtotal parathyroidectomy is preferred. (4). Another imperative consideration should be that many patients undergo prior total thyroidectomy, which warrants proper localization and special precaution during the surgery.

MULTIPLE ENDOCRINE NEOPLASIA (MEN) 4

Approximately 5–10% of patients with MEN-1 syndrome have alterations in genes other than *MEN1* gene, although there is no significant difference in their clinical manifestations. In these MEN1-like disorders about 3% are linked to one of eight known mutations to the CDNK1B gene, which encodes the 196 amino acid cyclin-dependent kinase inhibitor (CK1) p27^{kip1} located on chromosome 12p13. These mutations rarely found in patients with sporadic forms of PHPT (9).

HYPERPARATHYROIDISM-JAW TUMOR SYNDROME (HPT-JT)

HPT-JT is a rare autosomal dominant disorder characterized by the presence of PHPT due to a parathyroid adenoma or in some cases even parathyroid carcinoma, in addition to fibro-osseous jaw (maxilla and mandible) tumors, uterine tumors, and renal tumors. It is caused by a mutation in *CDC73/HRPT2* gene that encodes the protein parafibromin, presumed a tumor suppressor gene (3, 10, 11). PHPT is the first manifestation for most patients, with penetrance of more than 70%. The PHPT clinical course tends to be more aggressive and even life-threatening in comparison to sporadic or MEN-related disease. In addition, there is an unusually high rate of parathyroid carcinoma estimated in up to 10% of patients with HPT-JT. Most patients with *CDC73/HRPT2* mutations will develop PHPT around their late adolescence or early adulthood, and as early as the age of 7 for benign and 20 years for malignant parathyroid tumors. It has been suggested that screening for PHPT in patients with known mutations should start from age 5–10 (12–14). Mutations in the *CDC73/HRPT2* gene are found in 67–100% of parathyroid carcinoma, while rarely found in benign disease. It is recommended that these mutations should be tested in all cases of parathyroid carcinoma and in MEN1 mutations-negative patients with suspected familial PHPT (4, 14).

NON-SYNDROMIC CAUSES OF PRIMARY HYPERPARATHYROIDISM

Familial hypocalciuric hypercalcemia (FHH)

FHH is a lifelong benign cause of hypercalcemia which is inherited in a hetero-zygous autosomal dominant manner. It is caused by a loss of function mutation in the CaSR gene responsible for the calcium sensing receptor (CaSR) expressed on the parathyroid chief cells, kidney, and many other tissues. Decrease in its action causes "resetting" of the serum calcium concentration with elevated or inappropriately normal levels of PTH. In addition there is a PTH-independent low urinary calcium excretion. (12). The usual age of manifestation is during the neonatal period. These patients are usually asymptomatic, a fact that makes the estimation of its true prevalence very difficult. It is important to keep in mind this entity while evaluating a patient with hypercalcemia and PHPT since these patients do not require surgical intervention. Since biochemical and clinical parameters are often indistinguishable from PHPT, genetic testing could be help-ful in children with PHPT (14).

NEONATAL SEVERE HYPERPARATHYROIDISM (NSHPT)

NSHPT is an isolated form of PHPT found in neonates at birth or during their first 6 months of life, causing a severe symptomatic hypercalcemia. It results from a homozygous inactivation mutation to the CaSR gene (unlike heterozy-gous inactivation in FHH) leading to severe life-threatening hypercalcemia. NSHPT is characterized by severe hypercalcemia and hypophosphatemia, hypo-tonia, failure to thrive, bone demineralization secondary to osteoclast overactiv-ity with subsequent fractures, and respiratory difficulties secondary to ribcage involvement. This life-threatening disorder prompts urgent parathyroidectomy in order to correct their PTH-dependent hypercalcemia (3, 12, 15, 16).

REFERENCES

1. Press DM, Siperstein AE, Berber E, Shin JJ, Metzger R, Jin J, et al. The Prevalence of Undiagnosed and Unrecognized Primary Hyperparathyroidism: A Population-Based Analysis from the Electronic Medical Record. *Surgery* 2013;154(6):1232–8.

2. Kollars J, Zarroug AE, Heerden J Van, Lteif A, Stavlo P, Suarez L, et al. Primary Hyperparathyroidism in Pediatric Patients. *Pediatrics* 2005;115(4):974–80.
3. Thakker RV. Genetics of Parathyroid Tumours. *J Intern Med* 2016;280(6):574–83.
4. Wilhelm SM, Wang TS, Ruan DT, et al. The Definitive Management of Primary Hyperparathyroidism Who Needs an Operation? *JAMA* 2017;317(11):959–68.
5. Kamilaris CDC, Stratakis CA. Multiple Endocrine Neoplasia Type 1 (MEN1): An Update and the Significance of Early Genetic and Clinical Diagnosis. *Front Endocrinol (Lausanne)* 2019;10:1–15.
6. Norton JA, Krampitz G, Jensen RT. Multiple Endocrine Neoplasia Genetics and Clinical Management. *Surg Oncol Clin NA* 2015;24(4):795–832.
7. Men NT, Thakker RV, Newey PJ, Walls GV, Bilezikian J, Dralle H, et al. Clinical Practice Guidelines for Multiple Endocrine. *J Clin Endocrinol Metab* 2012;97(September):2990–3011.
8. Giri D, Mckay V, Weber A, Blair JC. Multiple Endocrine Neoplasia Syndromes 1 and 2 : Manifestations and Management in Childhood and Adolescence. *Arch Dis Child* 2015;100(10):994–9.
9. Thakker RV. Molecular and Cellular Endocrinology Multiple Endocrine Neoplasia type 1 (MEN1) and type 4 (MEN4). *Mol Cell Endocrinol* 2014;386(1–2):2–15.
10. Simonds WF, Branch MD, Diseases K. HHS Public Access. *Endocrinol Metab Clin North Am* 2017;46:405–18.
11. Mathews JW, Winchester R, Alsaygh N, Bartlett AM, Luttrell L. Hyperparathyroidism-Jaw Tumor Syndrome_ an Overlooked Cause of Severe Hypercalcemia. *Am J Med Sci* 2016;352(3):302–5.
12. Stokes VJ, Nielsen MF, Hannan FM, Thakker RV. Hypercalcemic Disorders in Children. *J Bone Miner Res* 2017;32(11):2157–70.
13. Starker LF, Åkerström T, Long WD, Delgado-Verdugo A, Donovan P, Udelsman R, et al. Frequent Germ-Line Mutations of the MEN1, CASR, and HRPT2 / CDC73 Genes in Young Patients with Clinically Non-Familial Primary Hyperparathyroidism. *Hormones Cancer* 2012;1(1–2):44–51.
14. Giusti F, Cavalli L, Cavalli T, Brandi ML. Hereditary Hyperparathyroidism Syndromes. *J Clin Densitom* 2013;16(1):69–74.
15. Davies JH, Shaw NJ. Investigation and Management of Hypercalcaemia in Children. *Arch Dis Child* 2012;97(6):533–8.
16. Falchetti A, Marini F, Giusti F, Cavalli L, Cavalli T, Brandi ML. DNA-Based Test : When and Why to Apply It to Primary Hyperparathyroidism Clinical Phenotypes *J Internal Med* 2009;266:69–83.

14

Hyperparathyroidism

KIMBERLY RAMONELL AND ERIN PARTINGTON BUCZEK

DIAGNOSIS

Hyperparathyroidism is defined as an elevated or inappropriately normal serum parathyroid hormone (PTH) level. Because PTH responds to calcium concentrations, the assessment of serum calcium is critical for determining the underlying etiology of HPT and appropriate classification of either primary, secondary, or tertiary HPT. Physical examination is often normal in HPT. Parathyroid glands are almost never palpable, even when enlarged, as they lie deep in the neck, posterior to the thyroid, and just medial to its lateral border. The role of laboratory evaluation and imaging studies are paramount in the diagnosis, preoperative assessment, and surgical planning of most patients with HPT and a comprehensive review of labs and imaging is detailed in other chapters.

ETIOLOGIES

Primary hyperparathyroidism

In conditions of high calcium levels, normal parathyroid glands respond to a negative feedback loop by decreasing their production and release of PTH, resulting in low serum PTH levels. However, in primary HPT, there is elevated or inappropriately normal PTH production in the setting of high serum calcium levels. The presence of these two biochemical derangements is diagnostic of classic primary HPT. However, Figure 14.1 summarizes the biochemical abnormalities that can differentiate the underlying etiologies of primary HPT even in the setting of inappropriately normal serum calcium and PTH levels.

Similar to adults, in the pediatric and adolescent populations, symptoms of primary HPT are related to the severity and duration of hypercalcemia. They are generally vague, can span the spectrum from mild to severe, and can be difficult to identify in young children. Common symptoms include abdominal pain, constipation, nausea and vomiting, pancreatitis, hematuria, uremia, polyuria, and peptic ulcers (2). Similar to adults, neuropsychiatric symptoms in children can manifest as mood swings, fatigue, depression, hypertension-related headaches, altered mental status, and coma (2). Primary HPT may also present with bone disease characterized by generalized demineralization and subperiosteal resorption, a characteristic feature of osteitis fibrosa cystica. Radiographically, this is most apparent on the radial aspect of the middle phalanx of the second or third fingers on hand X-rays. Brown tumors (osteoclastic tumors with a hemorrhagic component) and bone cysts occasionally develop. Disease severe enough to produce bone pain and pathologic fractures is rarely observed nowadays (3).

Children with primary HPT are more likely to be symptomatic at presentation when compared to adults and are more likely to have manifestations of end-organ damage at time of diagnosis. The reason for this discrepancy isn't completely understood but it is thought to be due in part to the prolonged delay in diagnosis in children (mean symptom duration was 24 months before diagnosis in a single large series) compared to adults who often undergo routine biochemical

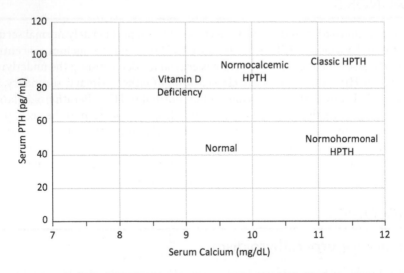

Figure 14.1 Primary hyperparathyroidism and variations in serum calcium and PTH levels to assist with identifying the presence of primary HPT even in the setting of normal serum calcium and normal serum PTH levels.

screening (1). Recent data suggest that there is a trend toward earlier diagnosis with an increase in the frequency of asymptomatic pediatric primary HPT presentations at a single institution from 56% to 79% over a 13-year period (4).

Primary HPT is the most common type of HPT in the pediatric population. Among children and adolescents with primary HPT, the most common etiology is a parathyroid adenoma. Similar to adults, the majority are single-gland disease with multiple adenomas being rare. Parathyroid adenomas develop due to somatic mutations in I-cells leading to clonal proliferation and excessive autologous PTH production, unresponsive to the hypercalcemia negative feedback loop (5). Parathyroid hyperplasia, characterized by multi-gland disease, is seen in up to 40% of sporadic primary HPT diagnoses in children versus only 10–15% in adults (1). Both children and adults with hereditary syndromes such as Multiple Endocrine Neoplasia (MEN) 1 and MEN2A are more likely to have four-gland hyperplasia than adenomatous disease. Table 14.1 summarizes the differential diagnosis of HPT.

A very rare and potentially lethal form of primary HPT that is unique to the pediatric population is neonatal severe primary hyperparathyroidism (NSHPT). NSHPT is due to an inherited homozygous loss-of-function mutation in the calcium sensing receptor (CaSR) gene (6). Neonates with NSHPT have complete absence, or severely attenuated function, of CaSR. This results in parathyroid hyperplasia, unregulated excessive PTH secretion, and severe hypercalcemia. NSHPT presents as early as the first few days of life with failure to thrive, hypotonia, and respiratory distress. Biochemical evaluation reveals markedly elevated, sometimes life-threatening hypercalcemia with serum calcium levels >20 mg/dL and severe metabolic bone disease. When evaluating the neonate

Table 14.1 Differential diagnosis of hyperparathyroidism

Type of hyperparathyroidism	Etiology
Primary	
	Parathyroid adenoma
	Parathyroid hyperplasia
	Parathyroid carcinoma
	Neonatal severe primary hyperparathyroidism
	Familial hypocalciuric hypercalcemia
	Genetic syndromes (MEN1, MEN2A, jaw-tumor)
Secondary	
	Chronic kidney disease
	1-α-hydroxylase deficiency
	Malabsorption/malnutrition
	Hereditary vitamin D-resistant rickets
Tertiary	
	Renal failure post-kidney transplant

with hypercalcemia, it is important to also rule out transient neonatal hyper-parathyroidism due to maternal hypocalcemia.

When only one allele is inactivated at this locus on the CaSR gene, the result is a milder and often asymptomatic form of primary HPT known as familial hypo-calciuric hypercalcemia (FHH). In FHH, PTH and calcium levels are usually only modestly elevated. The defining feature, hypocalciuria, occurs due to the impaired function of renally expressed CaSR which alters calcium reabsorption in the thick ascending limb (7). The presence of hypocalciuria (usually <100 mg/day) is protective against the development of nephrolithiasis and nephrocalcino-sis and helps distinguish FHH from other etiologies of primary HPT.

Genetic conditions associated with primary HPT in children and adolescents include MEN1, MEN2A, and hyperparathyroidism jaw-tumor syndrome, which are detailed in Chapter 13. Parathyroid adenocarcinoma is an exceptionally rare cause of primary HPT. It accounts for less than 1% of all cases of HPT in adults, and it is probably even more rare in children, although the exact incidence in the pediatric population is unknown (8). The diagnosis and management of parathy-roid cancer are reviewed in detail in Chapter 15.

Secondary hyperparathyroidism

Secondary HPT is a state of elevated PTH in the setting of low to normal serum calcium levels. Secondary HPT commonly occurs in patients with chronic renal failure but may also occur in those with hypocalcemia secondary to inadequate calcium or vitamin D intake or altered enteral malabsorption (Table 14.1). Vitamin D is essential to normal calcium homeostasis. Calcitriol is the activated form of vitamin D and increases intestinal calcium absorption. In vitamin D deficiency, there is inadequate substrate available for calcitriol production leading to reduced circulating calcitriol levels and insufficient intestinal calcium absorption, hypocalcemia, and resultant increased PTH production and bone resorption via osteoclast activation as a means to increase serum calcium levels (9).

Causes of vitamin D deficiency are numerous and include lack of production (due to lack of ultraviolet light exposure), inadequate oral intake, enteral malab-sorption, renal losses, and specific to the pediatric population, inborn errors of the 1-α-vitamin D hydroxylase gene which precludes normal calcitriol produc-tion. The pathophysiology of secondary HPT in chronic renal failure is complex and is related to hyperphosphatemia (and resultant hypocalcemia), deficiency of calcitriol due to loss of renal tissue, low calcium intake, decreased calcium absorption, and abnormal parathyroid cell response to extracellular calcium (9). The proximal renal tubule is the source of circulating calcitriol which is further reduced in patients with end-stage renal disease (ESRD).

All of these etiologies share a common pathophysiologic sequence: decreased calcium absorption results in a decrease in serum calcium levels, which is cor-rected by an appropriate increase in PTH and resultant bone calcium release.

Tertiary hyperparathyroidism

Tertiary HPT is rare in the pediatric population and occurs in the setting of prolonged parathyroid stimulation secondary to hypocalcemia, leading to parathyroid hyperplasia and subsequent autonomous PTH overproduction. Most commonly this occurs in patients with renal failure and secondary HPT who undergo renal transplant with restoration of kidney function. Despite the normalization of calcium homeostasis with renal transplantation, the autologous PTH production persists. Much like primary HPT, tertiary HPT presents with elevated serum calcium and elevated PTH levels. Biochemically they can sometimes be difficult to distinguish and rely on the medical history. The incidence has been reported to range from 0.5% to 5.6% of patients after renal transplant (10).

MANAGEMENT

The management of hyperparathyroidism in the pediatric population is largely extrapolated from adult guidelines. For primary HPT, the current NIH consensus guidelines, updated in 2014, recommend parathyroidectomy for all patients younger than 50 years of age with primary hyperparathyroidism, regardless of symptoms (11). Based on this, all children, adolescents, and young adults with primary HPT should undergo surgery. For preoperatively localized adenomas, a minimally invasive approach, defined as a 2-cm transverse collar incision, supplemented with the use of intra-operative PTH monitoring, is safe and highly curative in pediatric patients (12). Non-localizing or known multi-gland disease warrants a bilateral neck exploration. Four-gland hyperplasia is treated with either a total parathyroidectomy with auto-transplant (approximately 50 mg) or a subtotal (3.5 gland) parathyroidectomy with preservation of an adequate remnant size and cryopreservation of parathyroid tissue for possible auto-transplantation in the event of permanent postoperative hypoparathyroidism. The decision to choose subtotal versus total parathyroidectomy with auto-transplant for four-gland disease remains debatable and is detailed further in Chapter 16.

The indications for operative intervention in secondary HPT are not as well defined, particularly in the pediatric population. Medical treatment with calcium and vitamin D supplementation and administration of oral phosphate binders is usually successful in maintaining normal PTH and phosphorous levels in these patients but diet and medication compliance are critical. It is well-known that prolonged exposure to hyperphosphatemia, elevated PTH levels, and excessive bone loss lead to increased cardiovascular events and overall mortality in adults with ESRD, but the impact on the pediatric population is unknown (13). Early results from a pilot study using a single 0.25 mg/kg oral dose of cinacalcet, a calcimimetic that activates CaSR, in pediatric renal dialysis patients <6 years old showed promising results. Calcitriol lowered PTH by 30% at 8 hours post-administration, suggesting a potential role in the treatment of children with secondary HPT (14).

Similar to adults, surgical treatment of secondary HPT should be considered if the calcium phosphate product (Ca level × PO_4 level) is greater than 70 or if there is severe bone disease, uncontrolled pruritus, extensive soft tissue calcification with tumoral calcinosis, or calciphylaxis (15, 16). The operative approach to secondary HPT assumes four-gland hyperplasia and mandates bilateral exploration. If hyperplasia is present, a subtotal parathyroidectomy or a total parathyroidectomy with removal of all four glands and auto-transplantation of a small remnant in the forearm or neck muscle is performed (8).

In contrast to secondary HPT, the primary treatment of tertiary HPT is surgical. Among all tertiary HPT patients, 95–99% will have restoration of normal calcium homeostasis within 6 months post-renal transplant (10). In other words, while parathyroidectomy is the treatment for tertiary PTH, very few patients require surgery. Situations in which surgical treatment should be pursued include severe hypercalcemia defined as >11.5 mg/dL or persistent hypercalcemia of >10.2 mg/dL more than three months after transplant, concomitant severe osteopenia, renal calculi, or more classic symptoms of HPT including fatigue, pruritus, bone pain, pathologic bone fracture, peptic ulcer disease, or mental status changes (15).

SELECTED REFERENCES

1. Kollars J, Zarroug AE, van Heerden J, Lteif A, Stavlo P, Suarez L, et al. Primary Hyperparathyroidism in Pediatric Patients. *Pediatrics* 2005;115(4):974–80.
2. Markowitz M, Underland L, Gensure R. Parathyroid Disorders. *Pediatr Rev* 2016;37(12):524–35.
3. Allo M, Thompson NW, Harness JK, Nishiyama RH. Primary Hyperparathyroidism in Children, Adolescents, and Young Adults. *World J Surg* 1982;6(6):771–6.
4. Lou I, Schneider DF, Sippel RS, Chen H, Elfenbein DM. The Changing Pattern of Diagnosing Primary Hyperparathyroidism in Young Patients. *Am J Surg* 2017;213(1):146–50.
5. Williams RH. *Williams Textbook of Endocrinology*. Philadelphia, PA: Saunders; 2003.
6. Roizen J, Levine MA. Primary Hyperparathyroidism in Children and Adolescents. *J Chinese Med Assoc* 2012;75(9):425–34.
7. Moor M, Bonny O. Ways of Calcium Reabsorption in the Kidney. *Am J Renal Physiol* 2016;310(11):1337–50.
8. Burke J, Chen H, Gosain A. Parathyroid Surgery in Children. *Semin Pediatr Surg* 2014;23(2):66–70.
9. Lal G, Clark OH. Thyroid, Parathyroid, and Adrenal. In: Brunicardi F, Andersen DK, Billiar TR, et al. editors. *Schwartz's Principles of Surgery, 11e*. New York, NY: McGraw-Hill.
10. Dewberry LC Predictors of Tertiary Hyperparathyroidism: Who Will Benefit from Parathyroidectomy? *Surgery* 2014;156(6):1631–6.

11. Udelsman R, Åkerström G, Biagini C, Duh QY, Miccoli P, Niederle B, Tonelli F. The Surgical Management of Asymptomatic Primary Hyperparathyroidism: Proceedings of the Fourth International Workshop. *J Clin Endocrinol Metab* 2014;99(10):3595–606.

12. Mancilla EE, Levine MA, Adzick NS. Outcomes of Minimally Invasive Parathyroidectomy in Pediatric Patients with Primary Hyperparathyroidism Owing to Parathyroid Adenoma: A Single Institution Experience. *J Pediatr Surg* 2017;52(1):188–91.

13. Cozzolino M, Dusso AS, Slatopolsky E. Role of Calcium-Phosphate Product and Bone-Associated Proteins on Vascular Calcification in Renal Failure. *J Am Soc Nephrol* 2001;12(11):2511–6.

14. Sohn WY, Portale AA, Salusky IB, Zhang H, Yan LL, Ertik B, et al. An Open-Label, Single-Dose Study to Evaluate the Safety, Tolerability, Pharmacokinetics, and Pharmacodynamics of Cinacalcet in Pediatric Subjects Aged 28 Days to <6 Years with Chronic Kidney Disease Receiving Dialysis. *Pediatr Nephrol* 2019;34(1):145–54.

15. Pitt SC, Sippel RS, Chen H. Secondary and Tertiary Hyperparathyroidism, State of the Art Surgical Management. *Surg Clinics North Am* 2009;89(5):1227–39.

16. Madorin C, Owen RP, Fraser WD, Pellitteri PK, Radbill B, Rinaldo A, et al. The Surgical Management of Renal Hyperparathyroidism. *Eur Arch Otorhinolaryngology* 2012;269(6):1565–76.

15

Parathyroid carcinoma

JESSE T. DAVIDSON IV AND ALICIA DIAZ-THOMAS

PARATHYROID CANCER

In children, the diagnosis of parathyroid cancer is challenging and requires a multidisciplinary team evaluation with integration of all available data including clinical presentation, laboratory data, imaging, genetic testing, surgical evaluation, and histologic findings.

Clinical presentation

Initial risk assessment for parathyroid malignancy in adults is based on the severity of clinical presentation. The symptoms and sequelae, resulting from extreme hypercalcemia and hyperparathyroidism, are often constitutional (fatigue, depression, weight loss) with moderate to severe gastrointestinal disturbances (nausea, abdominal pain, vomiting, constipation). They may involve disease of the bone and kidney (polyuria, polydipsia, pathologic fracture, nephrolithiasis) or may be localized to the head and neck (dysphagia, palpable mass, neck pain, hoarseness, sore throat) (3). In the setting of benign primary hyperparathyroidism, adolescents tend to present with symptoms of hypercalcemia more commonly than adults (70–90% versus 20–50% of cases, respectively) (4). Therefore, benign and malignant disease in children may be indistinguishable based on symptom severity alone.

Laboratory data

Data on laboratory evaluation of pediatric parathyroid cancer are limited. In adult cases, serum calcium levels are markedly elevated at ≥13 mg/dL (5). PTH levels tend to be more varied, but elevations ≥3 times the upper limit of normal (≥195 pg/mL) are reported to be 84.4% sensitive and 80.0% specific for carcinoma (6). Among the few cases of pediatric parathyroid cancer reported in the literature, serum calcium levels ranged from 12.0 to 20.7 mg/dL, while PTH levels ranged from 190 to 8363 pg/mL (7, 8). In the adult population, the diagnosis of parathyroid cancer can be further evaluated by determining the third- to second-generation PTH ratio. Parathyroid cancer oversecretes amino PTH while benign parathyroid disease does not, and amino PTH is detected by third-, but not second-generation PTH assays. A ratio of >1 has a sensitivity of 81.8% and specificity of 97.3% for carcinoma (9, 10). This test has not been evaluated in children but may be a valuable diagnostic aid.

Imaging

To date, there is no dedicated imaging for parathyroid carcinoma *per se*. Imaging strategies follow guidelines for the localization of abnormal parathyroid glands in primary hyperparathyroidism. Preoperative evaluation can be achieved with neck ultrasound, contrasted CT of the neck and mediastinum, four-dimensional CT (4D-CT), planar sestamibi imaging, single photon emission CT (SPECT), SPECT/CT, or MRI. Imaging modality choice largely depends on availability of the technology, radiology expertise, and clinician preference. High-resolution neck ultrasound and planar sestamibi scintigraphy are the most commonly used studies to localize neoplastic parathyroid tissue in the preoperative setting (11). When malignancy is suspected, high-resolution anatomical studies (such as 4D-CT) can be useful to assess for invasion of surrounding structures, enlarged lymph nodes, or metastases. In addition, several CT findings have been associated with parathyroid cancer, including irregular shape, high short-to-long axis ratio, peritumoral infiltration, presence of calcifications, and low contrast enhancement (12). Additional evidence suggests that sestamibi imaging may be used to distinguish adenoma from carcinoma as well, as carcinoma tends to have higher retention levels of ^{99m}Tc-MIBI (13).

Genetic testing

Genetic testing is an essential tool in the diagnosis of pediatric parathyroid cancer. In particular, germline mutations and deletions in the transcription factor *CDC73* have been implicated in a spectrum of phenotypes, ranging from sporadic cases of parathyroid adenoma and carcinoma to Mendelian diseases such as hyperparathyroidism-jaw tumor syndrome (HPT-JT) and familial isolated hyperparathyroidism (FIHP) (14). HPT-JT and FIHP are autosomal dominant disorders that can give rise to parathyroid adenoma or carcinoma in childhood or early adulthood. HPT-JT may also present with fibro-osseous jaw tumors, cystic kidney lesions, and uterine fibromas. A careful family history is therefore critical. Some studies have reported that ~25% of HPT-JT patients may not harbor point mutations in the coding region or splice sites of the *CDC73* gene. Therefore, complete genetic testing must include methods to detect whole or partial deletions of the *CDC73* gene, or even mutations in the promoter, introns, or untranslated regions (UTRs) (14). If germline abnormalities in *CDC73* are found, referral to a genetic counselor is indicated.

Surgical evaluation

Adherence or infiltration of the parathyroid neoplasm to surrounding tissues at the time of resection has been used as an indicator of malignancy. If cancer is suspected, *en bloc* resection is indicated to achieve cure. Long-term survival rates have been reported at 89% with an 8% local recurrence rate for *en bloc* resection as compared with a 53% long-term survival and a 51% recurrence rate for simple parathyroidectomy alone (15). Risks for the development of distant metastases in adults include tumor size >3.2 cm, positive margins, nodal invasion, tumor rupture, and failure of intraoperative PTH to decrease after resection (16). Recurrent or metastatic disease is considered incurable and requires medical management.

Histological findings

Benign and malignant parathyroid neoplasia may be histologically indistinguishable. Parathyroid carcinoma has classically been described as having lobular architecture separated by fibrous bands, cytonuclear atypia, and mitoses (17), but these findings can be seen in benign disease as well. Vascular and capsular invasion are highly suggestive, but malignancy can only be confirmed by the presence or development of metastases (18). Loss of immunoreactivity of the CDC73 protein (also known as parafibromin) has also been associated with a higher probability of malignancy, but some parathyroid carcinomas continue to fully or partially express the protein, whereas a fraction of parathyroid adenomas demonstrates negative parafibromin staining (19). This variability has precluded its use as a routine tool in parathyroid cancer diagnosis, but it can add value as a component of a multifaceted evaluation. Differential expression of somatostatin receptors between parathyroid adenoma and carcinoma has been reported, and thus molecular characterization of tumors may hold promise in the development of individualized treatments (20).

Surveillance and management strategies for recurrent or metastatic parathyroid cancer

After surgical resection, surveillance for locoregional recurrence or distant metastases includes a history and physical with serum calcium levels every 6 months for the first year, annually for the next 2 years, then every other year. Patients should also undergo neck ultrasound annually. Follow-up should be lifelong as there is a risk of late recurrence (>10 years). Any abnormality found on surveillance necessitates detailed full-body imaging and biochemical evaluation (21). Once a patient has developed recurrent disease, surgical and medical management are palliative in nature. Subsequent locoregional surgical resection or distant metastatectomy can alleviate symptoms temporarily.

Management in recurrent disease focuses on medical agents to reduce symptoms and prolong life by mitigating hypercalcemia and its effects. Selective calcium-sensing receptor agonists (e.g., cinacalcet) and bisphosphonates are the primary treatment, but they tend to lose efficacy over time (22, 23). Denosumab, an antibody to the receptor activator of nuclear factor-KB ligand (RANKL) that blocks osteoclast development, has demonstrated considerable efficacy in managing hypercalcemia in adult parathyroid cancer (24) and thus may be a valuable palliative tool in children as well. Its use as a palliative agent in recurrent pediatric parathyroid cancer should be considered (authors' experience). Additionally, a recent adult case report suggests a chemotherapeutic agent, temozolomide, could also be considered as salvage therapy in tumors that express high O6-methylguanine DNA methyltransferase (MGMT) promoter methylation status, a known predictor of positive temozolomide treatment response in other tumors (25). Molecular profiling of parathyroid cancers can thus lead to identification of actionable therapeutic targets once other treatments have failed.

REFERENCES

1. Wei CH, Harari A. Parathyroid Carcinoma: Update and Guidelines for Management. *Curr Treat Options Oncol* 2012;13(1):11–23.
2. Fujimoto Y, Obara T, Ito Y, Kanazawa K, Aiyoshi Y, Nobori M. Surgical Treatment of Ten Cases of Parathyroid Carcinoma: Importance of an Initial En Bloc Tumor Resection. *World J Surg* 1984;8(3):392–8.
3. Levin KE, Galante M, Clark OH. Parathyroid Carcinoma Versus Parathyroid Adenoma in Patients with Profound Hypercalcemia. *Surgery* 1987;101(6):649–60.
4. Belcher R, Metrailer AM, Bodenner DL, Stack BC. Characterization of Hyperparathyroidism in Youth and Adolescents: A Literature Review. *Int J Pediatr Orl* 2013;77(3):318–22.
5. Shane E. Clinical Review 122: Parathyroid Carcinoma. *J Clin Endocrinol Metab* 2001;86(2):485–93.

6. Schaapveld M, Jorna FH, Aben KKH, Haak HR, Plukker JTM, Links TP. Incidence and Prognosis of Parathyroid Gland Carcinoma: A Population-Based Study in the Netherlands Estimating the Preoperative Diagnosis. *Am J Surg* 2011;202(5):590–7.

7. Davidson JT, Lam CG, McGee RB, Bahrami A, Diaz-Thomas A. Parathyroid Cancer in the Pediatric Patient. *J Pediatr Hematol Oncol* 2016;38(1):32–7.

8. Zivaljevic VR, Jovanovic MD, Djordjevic MS, Diklic AD, Paunovic IR. Case Report of Parathyroid Carcinoma in a Pediatric Patient. *Int J Pediatr Otorhinolaryngol* 2019;124:120–3.

9. Caron P, Maiza JC, Renaud C, Cormier C, Barres BH, Souberbielle JC. High Third Generation/Second Generation PTH Ratio in a Patient with Parathyroid Carcinoma: Clinical Utility of Third Generation/Second Generation PTH Ratio in Patients with Primary Hyperparathyroidism. *Clin Endocrinol (Oxf)* 2009;70(4):533–8.

10. Cavalier E, Daly AF, Betea D, Pruteanu-Apetrii PN, Delanaye P, Stubbs P, et al. The Ratio of Parathyroid Hormone as Measured by Third- And Second-Generation Assays as a Marker for Parathyroid Carcinoma. *J Clin Endocrinol Metab* 2010;95(8):3745–9.

11. Zafereo M, Yu J, Angelos P, Brumund K, Chuang HH, Goldenberg D, et al. American Head and Neck Society Endocrine Surgery Section Update on Parathyroid Imaging for Surgical Candidates with Primary Hyperparathyroidism. *Head Neck* 2019;41(7):2398–409.

12. Takumi K, Fukukura Y, Hakamada H, Nagano H, Kumagae Y, Arima H, et al. CT Features of Parathyroid Carcinomas: Comparison with Benign Parathyroid Lesions. *Jpn J Radiol* 2019;37(5):380–387.

13. Zhang M, Sun L, Rui W, Guo R, He H, Miao Y, et al. Semi-Quantitative Analysis of 99mTc-Sestamibi Retention Level for Preoperative Differential Diagnosis of Parathyroid Carcinoma. *Quant Imaging Med Surg* 2019;9(8):1394–401.

14. Newey PJ, Bowl MR, Cranston T, Thakker RV. Cell Division Cycle Protein 73 Homolog (CDC73) Mutations in the Hyperparathyroidism-Jaw Tumor Syndrome (HPT-JT) and Parathyroid Tumors. *Hum Mutat* 2010;31(3):295–307.

15. Koea JB, Shaw JHF. Parathyroid Cancer: Biology and Management. *Surg Oncol* 1999;8(3):155–65.

16. Asare EA, Silva-Figueroa A, Hess KR, Busaidy N, Graham PH, Grubbs EG, et al. Risk of Distant Metastasis in Parathyroid Carcinoma and its Effect on Survival: A Retrospective Review from a High-Volume Center. *Ann Surg Oncol* 2019;26(11):3593–9.

17. Schantz A, Castleman B. Parathyroid Carcinoma. A Study of 70 Cases. *Cancer* 1973;31(3):600–5.

18. Rodriguez C, Nadéri S, Hans C, Badoual C. Parathyroid Carcinoma: A Difficult Histological Diagnosis. *Eur Ann Otorhinolaryngol Head Neck Dis* 2012;129(3):157–9.

19. Juhlin CC, Höög A. Parafibromin as a Diagnostic Instrument for Parathyroid Carcinoma-Lone Ranger or Part of the Posse? *Int J Endocrinol* 2010;2010. https://doi.org/10.1155/2010/324964

20. Storvall S, Leijon H, Ryhänen E, Louhimo J, Haglund C, Schalin-Jäntti C, Arola J. Somatostatin Receptor Expression in Parathyroid Neoplasms. *Endocr Connect* 2019;8(8):1213–23.

21. Asare EA, Perrier ND. ASO Author Reflections: Distant Metastatic Parathyroid Carcinoma—Has the "Train Left the Station?" *Ann Surg Oncol* 2019;26(11):3600–1.

22. Marcocci C, Chanson P, Shoback D, Bilezikian J, Fernandez-Cruz L, Orgiazzi J, et al. Cinacalcet Reduces Serum Calcium Concentrations in Patients with Intractable Primary Hyperparathyroidism. *J Clin Endocrinol Metab* 2009;94(8):2766–72.

23. Szmuilowicz ED, Utiger RD. A Case of Parathyroid Carcinoma with Hypercalcemia Responsive to Cinacalcet therapy. *Nat Clin Pract Endocrinol Metab* 2006;2(5):291–6.

24. Vellanki P, Lange K, Elaraj D, Kopp PA, Muayed M El. Denosumab for Management of Parathyroid Carcinoma-Mediated Hypercalcemia. *J Clin Endocrinol Metab* 2014;99(2):387–90.

25. Storvall S, Ryhänen E, Bensch FV, Heiskanen I, Kytölä S, Ebeling T, et al. Recurrent Metastasized Parathyroid Carcinoma-Long-Term Remission After Combined Treatments with Surgery, Radiotherapy, Cinacalcet, Zoledronic acid, and Temozolomide. *JBMR Plus* 2019;3(4):e10114.

16

Parathyroid surgery in children

RAJSHRI M. GARTLAND, JESSICA FAZENDIN, AND
HERBERT CHEN

While parathyroid disease in children is rare, timely diagnosis and treatment are paramount for optimal childhood development. Indications for parathyroidectomy in children include primary hyperparathyroidism including for a single adenoma (most common), multiple endocrine neoplasia associated primary hyperparathyroidism, and neonatal severe primary hyperparathyroidism; secondary hyperparathyroidism in the setting of calcium phosphate product >70, severe bone disease, uncontrolled pruritus, extensive soft tissue calcification with calcinosis, and/or calciphylaxis; and tertiary hyperparathyroidism after renal transplantation in the setting of severe hypercalcemia (>11.5 mg/dL), persistent hypercalcemia (calcium >10.2 mg/dL for more than 3 months after transplant), severe osteopenia, renal calculi, PTH >400 pg/mL, and/or symptoms of primary hyperparathyroidism. Preoperative testing for an underlying familial cause, chiefly multiple endocrine neoplasia type 1, can facilitate operative planning and screening for other neoplastic processes. Depending on the patient's history and preoperative imaging studies, surgical options include minimally invasive parathyroidectomy and bilateral four-gland exploration. Video-assisted and endoscopic parathyroidectomy techniques have not been widely used or studied in children. Technical aspects of minimally invasive parathyroidectomy and bilateral parathyroid exploration, as well as postoperative care and outcomes, are outlined in this chapter.

TECHNIQUE

Minimally invasive parathyroidectomy

When preoperative imaging localizes an abnormal gland in a child with primary hyperparathyroidism, minimally invasive parathyroidectomy (MIP) can be considered. Compared to bilateral four-gland exploration, MIP involves a focused unilateral exploration. When performed in appropriate patients, MIP can be associated with shorter operative time, decreased risk of postoperative hypocalcemia, and less scarring on the contralateral side, making future neck surgery more feasible. In addition, while adults with primary hyperparathyroidism have been shown to have a slightly higher long-term recurrence rate with MIP compared to traditional bilateral exploration, this has not been reported in children with positive preoperative localization studies who undergo MIP.

The patient is positioned supine on the operative table with arms tucked and the neck gently extended. Most surgeons perform parathyroid surgery with general anesthesia while some may use local anesthesia with a deep cervical nerve block and sedation. A nerve-monitoring device may or may not be used. Prior to beginning the operation, a sample of peripheral blood is drawn in order to obtain a baseline pre-incision parathyroid hormone (PTH) value. The neck is then prepped with sterile solution and draped.

An approximately 2-cm transverse incision is made in a skin crease below the cricoid and above the sternal notch at either the midline or to the side of planned exploration. A surgeon-performed ultrasound after positioning may aid with the decision about incision placement. Electrocautery is used to incise through the platysma. The strap muscles are identified and separated longitudinally along the median raphe to expose the thyroid. The strap muscles are then elevated laterally away from the anterior surface of the thyroid gland and the thyroid lobe elevated medially on the side of the localized parathyroid gland for exposure. An enlarged superior parathyroid gland is usually seen on the undersurface of the upper half of the thyroid gland posterior and lateral to the recurrent laryngeal nerve, whereas an enlarged inferior parathyroid gland is usually located anterior to the recurrent laryngeal nerve and caudal to the inferior thyroid artery near the lower half of the thyroid lobe. Circumferential dissection of the gland is performed while avoiding grasping or fracturing the gland, and the venous tributary and artery of the gland are clipped and divided before gland excision.

After excision, a post-excision PTH value is drawn. As PTH has a half-life of 3–7 minutes, a PTH decline of >50% after 5, 10, and/or 15 minutes suggests that an adequate amount of hyperfunctioning tissue has been removed. Failure of PTH levels to drop may suggest the need to convert to a bilateral exploration. The interpretation of intraoperative PTH monitoring can be more challenging in patients with pre-incision PTH levels <100, or in patients with renal failure effecting normal clearance of PTH. Intraoperative PTH monitoring has been shown to be an effective tool to confirm cure in pediatric patients, and pediatric patients can have a more dramatic drop in PTH levels compared to adults. Closure of the wound is then performed by reapproximating the strap muscles, platysma, and skin, and applying a sterile dressing.

Bilateral four-gland exploration

The patient is positioned, prepped, and draped, and a pre-incision PTH is drawn in a similar fashion as for the minimally invasive parathyroidectomy approach above. A transverse incision, usually no greater than 4 cm, is made in a natural skin crease below the cricoid and above the sternal notch. The strap muscles are identified and separated longitudinally along the median raphe to expose the thyroid. The strap muscles are then elevated laterally away from the anterior surface of the thyroid gland and the thyroid lobe elevated medially on the first side. With the lateral and posterior surface of the thyroid exposed, the middle thyroid vein may come into view and can be ligated to facilitate further exposure. Exposure of the superior parathyroid gland involves more medial rotation of the thyroid gland and identifying the fatty tissue adjacent to where branches of the superior and inferior thyroid artery enter the thyroid.

Staying close to the thyroid during dissection will help prevent inadvertent injury to the recurrent laryngeal nerve; while the recurrent laryngeal nerve does not need to be skeletonized during parathyroid exploration, consideration of its path in relation to the parathyroid can help facilitate a safe dissection. Abnormal or enlarged glands often appear as a sliding bulge beneath a veil of overlying tissue. Once the gland is identified, the remaining ipsilateral parathyroid gland can be explored next, followed by the glands on the contralateral side.

Once all parathyroid glands have been identified, a decision can be made regarding the extent of parathyroidectomy based on the suspected disease process (single adenoma versus double adenoma versus four-gland hyperplasia). If only some of the parathyroid glands are abnormal, the abnormal glands can be dissected free and excised, while the remaining normal gland(s) can be left in situ and marked with a clip. Four-gland hyperplasia is typically treated with subtotal parathyroidectomy, resecting all glands except for a remnant the size of a normal parathyroid gland, or with total parathyroidectomy and auto-transplantation. Inferior parathyroid glands are best used as remnants if otherwise suitable given that they are more easily accessed in the setting of reoperation. Cryopreservation of excised parathyroid issue can also be utilized but many studies have shown that this is not very effective. When four glands are identified but the PTH remains elevated, there may be a supernumerary parathyroid gland, often found in the cervical thymus. If both tracks of the cervical thymus do not reveal a supernumerary parathyroid gland, additional postoperative imaging, and potentially selective venous sampling may be necessary and most appropriate before pursuing further exploration.

When initial exploration fails to reveal all four glands, several spaces can be further evaluated including the retroesophageal space, the cervical thymus, high or deep parapharyngeal or paratracheal spaces, or the carotid sheath. An intrathyroidal parathyroid gland may require enucleation or thyroid lobectomy. Using a systematic approach to find ectopic glands is particularly important given that up to 25% of pediatric patients with primary hyperparathyroidism can have an ectopic gland compared to 6–16% of adult patients. After exploration and resection are completed, an intraoperative PTH level can be obtained, with wound closure to follow, as outlined in the "Minimally invasive parathyroidectomy" section, if the PTH level indicates that an adequate amount of hyperfunctioning tissue has been removed.

Radio-guided parathyroidectomy in children

Radio-guided parathyroidectomy involves intravenous injection of technetium-99m sestamibi 1–2 hours preoperatively and then use of a gamma probe intraoperatively to help localize hyperfunctioning parathyroid glands (Figure 16.1). After the gland is removed, a radionucleotide count greater than 20% of background indicates adequate removal of hyperfunctioning parathyroid tissue. This technique has proven successful in identifying hyperfunctional parathyroid tissue in pediatric patients, despite smaller gland sizes, with equal cure rates in

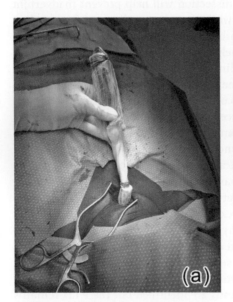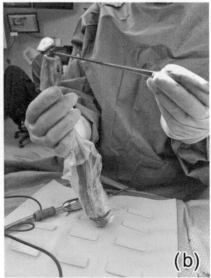

Figure 16.1 Use of radio-guidance for the confirmation of abnormal parathyroid glands. The gamma probe is placed over the thyroid to obtain a background count (**A**). An abnormal gland is identified and resected and then placed on the probe to obtain an ex-vivo count. The parathyroid is confirmed abnormal if the count is ≥20% of the background count (**B**).

pediatric and adult populations. Radio-guidance can be particularly helpful in guiding exploration of ectopic glands.

POSTOPERATIVE CARE

Postoperatively, patients are monitored for signs of hematoma, voice changes, and hypocalcemia. Pediatric patients, like adults, can often be discharged home the same day if they have minimal co-morbidities and if the operation was uneventful. Younger children who cannot reliably report symptoms can be observed overnight. There are generally no restrictions on diet or activity, and patients are discharged with calcium supplements to be used as needed. Patients who undergo total parathyroidectomy with auto-transplant require both calcium and calcitriol replacement at discharge since the autograft can take at least 2 weeks to become functional. Children who undergo parathyroidectomy for hyperparathyroidism require lifelong monitoring for symptoms of recurrent hypercalcemia.

OUTCOMES OF PARATHYROIDECTOMY IN CHILDREN

Patients are deemed "cured" after parathyroidectomy if they are able to maintain normal calcium levels over the long term. Pediatric patients experience cure rates of 96–100% after parathyroidectomy for hyperparathyroidism, rates similar to the adult population. In children with chronic kidney disease, total parathyroidectomy with auto-transplantation provides excellent long-term control of hyperparathyroidism and calcium-phosphate metabolism, and may thus mitigate cardiovascular-related disease and uremic bone disease.

Recurrent hyperparathyroidism refers to normalization of calcium levels after parathyroidectomy but then a return of high calcium levels >6 months postoperatively. While rare, recurrent hyperparathyroidism is more common in the setting of familial disease, and carries a higher risk of the diseased gland being in an ectopic location. Reoperative surgery in this setting carries an increased risk of complications, and both preoperative vocal cord assessment and use of intraoperative adjuncts such as intraoperative PTH monitoring, radio-guidance, and/or intraoperative nerve monitoring should be considered in this setting.

The main complications after parathyroidectomy include bleeding, infection, unilateral or bilateral recurrent laryngeal nerve injury, and hypoparathyroidism and hypocalcemia. Multiple studies have demonstrated that children are at higher risk of general and endocrine-specific complications after parathyroidectomy compared to adults, and that this risk is related to both pre-existing kidney disease and to age, with more complications occurring in younger children. In light of this increased risk of postoperative complications in the pediatric population, as well as the increased rate of ectopic parathyroid adenomas in children, children undergoing parathyroidectomy benefit from multi-specialty care that includes the expertise of high-volume endocrine surgeons.

SELECTED REFERENCES

Burke JF, Chen H, Gosain A. Parathyroid Surgery in Children. *Semin Pediatr Surg* 2014;23(2):66–70.

Burke JF, Jacobson K, Gosain A, Sippel RS, Chen H. Radioguided Parathyroidectomy Effective in Pediatric Patients. *J Surg Res* 2013;184(1):312–7.

Dream S, Wang R, Lovell K, Iyer P, Lindeman B, Chen H. Outpatient thyroidectomy in the pediatric population. *Am J Surg* 2020; 219(6): 890–3.

Durkin ET, Nichol PF, Lund DP, Chen H, Sippel RS. What is the Optimal Treatment for Children with Primary Hyperparathyroidism? *J Pediatr Surg* 2010;45(6):1142–6.

Kollars J, Zarroug AE, van Heerden J, Lteif A, Stavlo P, Suarez L, et al. Primary Hyperparathyroidism in Pediatric Patients. *Pediatrics* 2005;115(4):974–80.

Mancilla EE, Levine MA, Adzick NS. Outcomes of Minimally Invasive Parathyroidectomy in Pediatric Patients with Primary Hyperparathyroidism Due to Parathyroid Adenoma: A Single Institution Experience. *J Pediatr Surg* 2017;52(1):188–91.

Pitt SC, Sippel RS, Chen H. Secondary and Tertiary Hyperparathyroidism, State of the Art Surgical Management. *Surg Clin North Am* 2009;89(5):1227–39.

Rampp RD, Mancilla EE, Adzick NS, Levine MA, Kelz RR, Fraker DL, et al. Single Gland, Ectopic Location: Adenomas are Common Causes of Primary Hyperparathyroidism in Children and Adolescents. *World J Surg* 2020;44(5):1518–1525.

Romero Arenas MA, Morris LF, Rich TA, Cote GJ, Grubbs EG, Waguespack SG, Perrier ND. Preoperative Multiple Endocrine Neoplasia Type 1 Diagnosis Improves the Surgical Outcomes of Pediatric Patients with Primary Hyperparathyroidism. *J Pediatr Surg* 2014;49(4):546–50.

Schaefer B, Schlosser K, Wuhl E, Schall P, Klaus G, Schaefer F, Schmitt CP. Long-Term Control of Parathyroid Hormone and Calcium-Phosphate Metabolism After Parathyroidectomy in Children with Chronic Kidney Disease. *Nephrol Dial Transplant* 2010;25(8):2590–5.

Schlosser K, Schmitt CP, Bartholomaeus JE, Suchan KL, Buchler MW, Rothmund M, Weber T. Parathyroidectomy for Renal Hyperparathyroidism in Children and Adolescents. *World J Surg* 2008;32(5):801–6.

Sosa JA, Tuggle CT, Wang TS, Thomas DC, Boudourakis L, Rivkees S, Roman SA. Clinical and Economic Outcomes of Thyroid and Parathyroid Surgery in Children. *J Clin Endocrinol Metab* 2008;93(8):3058–65.

Tuggle CT, Roman SA, Wang TS, Boudourakis L, Thomas DC, Udelsman R, Ann Sosa J. Pediatric Endocrine Surgery: Who is Operating on our Children? *Surgery* 2008;144(6):869–77.

Index

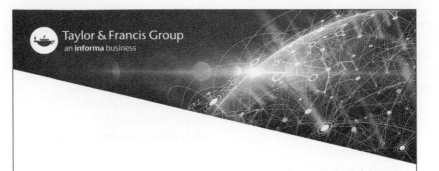

Printed and bound by CPI Group (UK) Ltd, Croydon, CR0 4YY

23/10/2024

01778263-0010